Psychiatric Care in Primary Care Practice

Editor

JANET R. ALBERS

PRIMARY CARE: CLINICS IN OFFICE PRACTICE

www.primarycare.theclinics.com

Consulting Editor
JOEL J. HEIDELBAUGH

June 2016 • Volume 43 • Number 2

ELSEVIER

1600 John F. Kennedy Boulevard ● Suite 1800 ● Philadelphia, Pennsylvania, 19103-2899

http://www.theclinics.com

PRIMARY CARE: CLINICS IN OFFICE PRACTICE Volume 43, Number 2
June 2016 ISSN 0095-4543, ISBN-13: 978-0-323-44630-3

Editor: Jessica McCool
Developmental Editor: Colleen Viola

Primary Care: Clinics in Office Practice (ISSN: 0095–4543) is published quarterly by Elsevier Inc., 360 Park Avenue South, New York, NY 10010-1710. Months of issue are March, June, September, and December. Periodicals postage paid at New York, NY and additional mailing offices. Subscription prices are $225.00 per year (US individuals), $434.00 (US institutions), $100.00 (US students), $275.00 (Canadian individuals), $491.00 (Canadian institutions), $175.00 (Canadian students), $345.00 (international individuals), $491.00 (international institutions), and $175.00 (international students). Foreign air speed delivery is included in all *Clinics* subscription prices. All prices are subject to change without notice. POSTMASTER: Send address changes to *Primary Care: Clinics in Office Practice*, Elsevier Periodicals Customer Service, 11830 Westline Industrial Drive, St. Louis, MO 63146. Customer Service Health Sciences Division, Subscription Customer Service, 3251 Riverport Lane, Maryland Heights, MO 63043. **Customer Service: 1-800-654-2452 (U.S. and Canada); 314-447-8871 (outside U.S. and Canada). Fax: 314-447-8029. E-mail: journalscustomerservice-usa@elsevier.com (for print support); journalsonlinesupport-usa@elsevier.com (for online support).**

Reprints. For copies of 100 or more, of articles in this publication, please contact the Commercial Reprints Department, Elsevier Inc., 360 Park Avenue South, New York, NY 10010-1710. Tel. 212-633-3874; Fax: 212-633-3820; E-mail: reprints@elsevier.com.

Primary Care: Clinics in Office Practice is covered in *MEDLINE/PubMed (Index Medicus)* and *EMBASE/ Excerpta Medica, Current Contents/Clinical Medicine, and ISI/BIOMED.*

Contributors

CONSULTING EDITOR

JOEL J. HEIDELBAUGH, MD, FAAFP, FACG
Clinical Professor, Departments of Family Medicine and Urology, Clerkship Director, Department of Family Medicine, University of Michigan Medical School, Ann Arbor, Michigan; Ypsilanti Health Center, Ypsilanti, Michigan

EDITOR

JANET R. ALBERS, MD, FAAFP
Professor and Chair, Department of Family and Community Medicine, Southern Illinois University School of Medicine, Springfield, Illinois

AUTHORS

CRISTIN S. ADAMS, DO
PGY-3 Trident/MUSC Family Medicine Residency, Department of Family Medicine, Medical University of South Carolina, Charleston, South Carolina

NORAH BAKER, MD
Physician, Red Bud Clinic Corporation, Red Bud, Illinois

JOSEPH J. BENICH III, MD
Assistant Professor, Department of Family Medicine, Medical University of South Carolina, Charleston, South Carolina

RUSSELL BLACKWELDER, MD, MDiv
Assistant Professor of Family Medicine, Medical University of South Carolina, Charleston, South Carolina

SCOTT W. BRAGG, PharmD
Assistant Professor, South Carolina College of Pharmacy (MUSC Campus), Department of Family Medicine, Medical University of South Carolina, Charleston, South Carolina

MELVANIA BRIGGS, MA, PA-C
Medical Instructor and Academic Coordinator, Physician Assistant Program, Department of Community and Family Medicine, Duke University School of Medicine, Durham, North Carolina

GENE COMBS, MD
Associate Clinical Professor, Departments of Family Medicine and Psychiatry, NorthShore University HealthSystem, Glenbrook Hospital, University of Chicago, Glenview, Illinois

ELIZABETH W. COZINE, MD
Instructor in Family Medicine, Department of Family Medicine, Mayo Clinic, Rochester, Minnesota

MARY IFTNER DOBBINS, MD
Associate Professor, Director, Mental Health Integration, Department of Family and Community medicine, SIU School of Medicine, Springfield, Illinois

DOROTHY DSCHIDA, MD
Northwestern McGaw Family Medicine Residency Program, Erie Family Heath Center, Chicago, Illinois

JOHN R. FREEDY, MD, PhD
Associate Professor of Family Medicine, Trident Family Medicine Residency, Department of Family Medicine, Medical University of South Carolina, Charleston, South Carolina

ROCHELLE F. HANSON, PhD
Professor, Department of Psychiatry and Behavioral Sciences, National Crime Victims Research and Treatment Center, Medical University of South Carolina, Charleston, South Carolina

SHARON K. HULL, MD, MPH
Professor and Division Chief, Family Medicine, Department of Community and Family Medicine, Duke University School of Medicine, Durham, North Carolina

STACY LEE, LCSW
SIU School of Medicine, Springfield, Illinois

BOBBY LEEBOLD, LCSW
Behavioral Instructor, Decatur Family Medicine Residency, Southern Illinois University School of Medicine, Decatur, Illinois

DAVID MAHONEY, MD, MBE
Mount Pleasant Family Practice, Roper St. Francis Physicians, Charleston, South Carolina

STACY L. STOKES MELTON, LCSW
SIU Center for Family Medicine, Quincy, Illinois

DANIELLE H. METZLER, MD
PGY3 Family Medical Resident, Trident Family Medicine Residency, Department of Family Medicine, Medical University of South Carolina, Charleston, South Carolina

THOMAS H. MILLER, MD
Program Director, SIU Quincy Family Medicine Residency, Associate Professor, Clinical Family and Community Medicine, SIU School of Medicine, Quincy, Illinois

LAUREN OSHMAN, MD, MPH
Assistant Clinical Professor, Department of Family Medicine, NorthShore University HealthSystem, Glenbrook Hospital, University of Chicago, Glenview, Illinois

KENYON RAILEY, MD
Assistant Professor, Physician Assistant Program, Department of Community and Family Medicine, Duke University School of Medicine, Durham, North Carolina

DEVDUTTA SANGVAI, MD, MBA
Associate Professor of Family Medicine, Pediatrics and Psychiatry, Duke University School of Medicine, Durham, North Carolina

MARY R. TALEN, PhD
Northwestern McGaw Family Medicine Residency Program, Erie Family Heath Center, Chicago, Illinois

JOHNNY C. TENEGRA, MD, MS
Assistant Professor, Decatur Family Medicine Residency, Southern Illinois University School of Medicine, Decatur, Illinois

SHEILA A. THOMAS, MD
SIU School of Medicine, Springfield, Illinois

DONNA TUCCERO, MD
Assistant Professor, Associate Family Medicine Residency Program Director, Department of Community and Family Medicine, Duke University School of Medicine, Durham, North Carolina

KRISTEN HOOD WATSON, MD
Assistant Professor of Family Medicine, Medical University of South Carolina, Charleston, South Carolina

SANTINA WHEAT, MD, MPH
Northwestern McGaw Family Medicine Residency Program, Erie Family Heath Center, Chicago, Illinois

JOHN M. WILKINSON, MD
Associate Professor of Family Medicine, Department of Family Medicine, Mayo Clinic, Rochester, Minnesota

ANDREW YOCHUM, DO
Assistant Professor, Department of Family Medicine, Southern Illinois University-Carbondale, Carbondale, Illinois

Contents

> The primary care medical home continues to adapt by applying new research to population health approaches to care. With the discovery that life experiences trigger a chain of biologic events linked to chronic illnesses, the role of patient-centered multidisciplinary care teams becomes of paramount importance. Subsequently, mental health professionals are being incorporated into the primary care setting, using their skills in nontraditional models to customize care for each patient. This "integration" of primary care and unique mental health services engenders opportunity for enhanced clinical care, professional workforce development and support, more effective population health initiatives, and informed health care policy.

> This article reviews the history, methodology, and evidence related to the effective use of motivational interviewing (MI) in the primary care setting. MI has been shown to have a positive effect in promotion and modification of health habits and to increase treatment engagement. MI is also effective when used in conjunction with other treatment modalities, such as educational programs and cognitive behavioral therapy. Practical application of MI can be accomplished in a variety of primary care settings by a wide range of practitioners, incorporates nicely into new health care delivery models, and may improve the patient-provider relationship.

> Chronic pain and its associated syndrome have become increasingly prevalent in primary care. With the increase in narcotic use and subsequent adverse events, primary care physicians often seek safer alternatives to treating this condition. Prescribing narcotics necessitates using methods to screen for high abuse risk and protect against misuse. With the understanding of how chronic pain is related to mental illnesses such as depression and posttraumatic stress disorder, mindfulness techniques and

behavioral therapy can be used to help decrease the dependence on dangerous opioid medications and help patients understand, accept, and cope with their chronic pain.

One of the more prevalent and often undiagnosed problems seen by primary care clinicians is substance misuse. Resulting in increased morbidity and mortality, loss of productivity, and increased health care costs, substance misuse in our society remains a significant public health issue. Primary care physicians are on the front lines of medical care, and as such, are in a distinctive position to recognize potential problems in this area and assist. This article outlines office-based screening approaches and strategies for managing and treating this complex issue confronting primary care.

This article focuses on six basic components of more effective depression care, emphasizing systems of team-based and collaborative care for diagnosis, monitoring, and follow-up. It also emphasizes the principles of stepped care and proactive and timely intensification of treatment, and discusses various augmentation strategies that all primary care providers could more readily employ.

Investigation for a possible anxiety disorder should be considered in patients with multiple or persistent anxiety symptoms or multiple somatic complaints without a clear somatic etiology. The ideal treatment for anxiety disorders is a combination of pharmacologic and behavioral strategies. As primary care health care evolves, it is expected that the management of mental health disorders (including anxiety disorders) will largely occur in the context of collaborative care models in which patients and primary care clinicians are assisted by trained case managers who help facilitate a more comprehensive, holistic treatment plan between primary care and mental health providers.

Personality disorders are a group of diagnostic categories applicable when people show personality traits that are so extreme they cause clear difficulties in their lives and relationships. More widespread agreement is found on sorting by three broad categories (odd/eccentric, dramatic/emotional/erratic, and anxious/fearful) than by more specific subtypes. Primary care physicians need to recognize when extreme personality traits are causing difficulties in their relationships with patients and to have a way to approach these difficulties when they arise. This article reviews current thinking on the diagnosis and treatment of personality disorders, focusing especially on dramatic/emotional/erratic disorders, which are those most often problematic in clinical settings.

Bipolar Disorder   269
Thomas H. Miller

Bipolar disorder is a chronic mental health disorder that is frequently encountered in primary care. Many patients with depression may actually have bipolar disorder. The management of bipolar disorder requires proper diagnosis and awareness or referral for appropriate pharmacologic therapy. Patients with bipolar disorder require primary care management for comorbidities such as cardiovascular and metabolic disorders.

Autism Spectrum/Pervasive Developmental Disorder   285
Andrew Yochum

Autism spectrum disorder is a complex disorder that is becoming more prevalent. Because of this increased prevalence, primary care providers must become more knowledgeable about the disorder so they can provide appropriate screening, evaluation, and treatment as part of an interdisciplinary team and to serve patients and families within the medical home.

Eating Disorders in the Primary Care Setting   301
Devdutta Sangvai

Eating disorders are a complex set of illnesses most commonly affecting white adolescent girls and young women. The most common eating disorders seen in the primary care setting are anorexia nervosa, bulimia nervosa, and binge eating disorder. Treatment in the primary care environment ideally involves a physician, therapist, and nutritionist, although complex cases may require psychiatric and other specialist care. Early diagnosis and treatment are associated with improved outcomes, whereas the consequences of untreated eating disorders, particularly anorexia nervosa, can be devastating, including death.

Childhood Sexual Abuse: Identification, Screening, and Treatment Recommendations in Primary Care Settings   313
Rochelle F. Hanson and Cristin S. Adams

It is estimated that 8% to 12% of American youths have experienced at least one sexual assault in their lifetime, making childhood sexual abuse (CSA) an important public health problem that is likely to be encountered by primary care providers. Use of screening tools and understanding the principles behind targeted clinical evaluation can aid in identification of CSA victims despite highly variable presentation. The primary care provider must be aware of potential signs and symptoms as well as differential diagnoses in order to identify children who may benefit from further mental health evaluation and intervention.

PRIMARY CARE:
CLINICS IN OFFICE PRACTICE

THE CLINICS ARE AVAILABLE ONLINE!
Access your subscription at:
www.theclinics.com

Foreword

Objectivity and Compassion

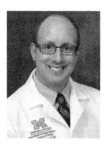

Joel J. Heidelbaugh, MD, FAAFP, FACG
Consulting Editor

One of my third-year medical students recently commented, "Why do you see so much psych in your practice? Why don't you just refer all of these patients with depression, anxiety, and stress to a psychiatrist"? The same student later commented, "I'm impressed that you spent time motivating your patient to take better care of himself in managing his diabetes and metabolic syndrome—*when do we learn those techniques in medical school*"?

As in many of my previous forewords for the *Primary Care: Clinics in Office Practice* series, I have stated the challenges of teaching the necessary tools and knowledge to address many complex medical and psychosocial issues within 4 years of medical school and 3 years of primary care residency. While this continues to be a formidable challenge, the proverbial bar becomes raised even higher day after day in meeting the needs of our patients—without simply referring our patients to a specialist when we can be well equipped to diagnose and treat common psychiatric conditions. Appropriate psychiatric treatment requires longitudinal care, sequential assessments, hours of compassionate listening, and the ability to motivate people to make positive changes in their lives. Primary care providers are poised to accept this challenge.

This issue of *Primary Care: Clinics in Office Practice* dedicated to psychiatric care in the primary care setting highlights many salient components of psychiatric care requisite for daily practice. The issue commences with detailing the important conceptual framework of how psychiatric care is integrated through multidisciplinary teams, a necessary construct to understand and utilize relative to our resources. Articles outlining motivational interviewing techniques, cognitive behavioral therapy, and mindfulness techniques contain strategies that clinicians can easily implement and teach that will improve outcomes. Many of the common psychiatric diagnoses seen in primary care are explored in detail, including depression, anxiety, bipolar disorder, personality disorders, autism spectrum disorders, and psychiatric emergencies. A dedicated article highlighting pharmacotherapy is rich in practical information that is always evolving.

Prim Care Clin Office Pract 43 (2016) xiii–xiv
http://dx.doi.org/10.1016/j.pop.2016.03.002
0095-4543/16/$ – see front matter © 2016 Published by Elsevier Inc.

primarycare.theclinics.com

We are experiencing a significant paucity of medical students and residents who will build their careers on managing patients with substance abuse disorders as well as treating children and adolescents with psychiatric disorders. The rates of autism spectrum disorders have become alarmingly high, with limited resources in our communities and schools to properly treat, guide, and educate these children.

I would like to offer my gratitude to Dr Janet Albers and her colleagues for their substantial efforts in creating yet another unique and highly practical compendium of articles that are information-rich and easily adaptable to daily primary care practice. Perhaps most impressively poignant is the final article, dedicated to physician wellness across the professional spectrum. When we can appropriately mind our own mental health, we can then best help our patients through objectivity and compassion.

Joel J. Heidelbaugh, MD, FAAFP, FACG
Departments of Family Medicine and Urology
University of Michigan Medical School
Ann Arbor, MI 48109, USA

Ypsilanti Health Center
200 Arnet Suite 200
Ypsilanti, MI 48198, USA

E-mail address:
jheidel@umich.edu

Preface

Integrating Psychiatric Care into Primary Care Practice

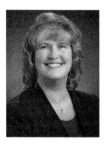

Janet R. Albers, MD
Editor

For too many years, mental health and physical health have been addressed in separate silos within the health care system. Due to stigma, many patients suffering with mental health issues are never diagnosed or treated. By integrating the care of mental and behavioral health into the patient-centered medical home, outcomes are greatly improved. Due to time constraints and discomfort with content, many primary care providers find it difficult to address these important issues. An integrated care team—including primary care physicians, nurses, advanced practice professionals, behavioral health providers (licensed clinical professional counselor, licensed clinical social worker, clinical psychologists), psychiatrists, care coordinators/case managers, and clinical pharmacists, to name a few—is better able to promote health and screen for, diagnose, and treat the whole patient in an efficient and effective way. Patients welcome the accessibility and comfort of this care within their trusted medical home.

My hope is that this issue of "Psychiatric Care in Primary Care Practice" will serve as a practical tool for excellent care of the patient. From the expanding role of the integrated interdisciplinary team to the use of motivational interviewing as part of the treatment of chronic illnesses to the care of the chronic pain patient and those with substance abuse issues, this serves as a resource that is usable for the primary care clinician in practice or the medical student or resident in training. Common mental health diagnoses, such as depression, anxiety, personality, and bipolar disorders, are included, as well as specific articles on autism spectrum disorders, eating disorders, and child sexual abuse. An article on psychopharmacology and one on psychiatric emergencies round out the issue, which closes with an extremely relevant article on physician wellness as a crucial element of the "Quadruple Aim": better health, better health care, lower cost, and wellness/satisfaction of the health care

Prim Care Clin Office Pract 43 (2016) xv–xvi
http://dx.doi.org/10.1016/j.pop.2016.03.001
0095-4543/16/$ – see front matter © 2016 Published by Elsevier Inc.

team. Please use this issue as a means to expand your comfort in caring for the whole patient, including psychiatric and behavioral issues, which are so fundamental to overall health.

Janet R. Albers, MD
Department of Family
and Community Medicine
Southern Illinois University School of Medicine
PO Box 19670
520 North 4th Street
Springfield, IL 62702, USA

E-mail address:
jalbers@siumed.edu

Integrated Care and the Evolution of the Multidisciplinary Team

Mary Iftner Dobbins, MD[a],*, Sheila A. Thomas, MD[a],
Stacy L. Stokes Melton, LCSW[b], Stacy Lee, LCSW[a]

KEYWORDS

- Integrated care • Behavioral health • Health care teams • Primary care psychiatry
- Workforce development

KEY POINTS

- Primary care practice in the patient-centered medical home is transforming as new findings are considered in the context of population health and changes driven by health care reform.
- Research in neuroscience, epigenetics, human development, trauma-informed care, and population health describes the biologic chain of events linking life experiences with chronic medical and mental illnesses.
- Mental health professionals are increasingly being incorporated into the medical home as part of a team approach to the provision of care.
- These professionals use their skills in nontraditional models to customize care for each patient as indicated, creating an expanded definition of their specialty.
- "Integration" of primary care and mental health services engenders opportunity for enhanced clinical care, professional workforce development and support, more effective population health initiatives, and informed health care policy.

INTRODUCTION
Patient-Centered Care

Primary care disciplines continue to contribute a unique and vital perspective to the practice of medicine. Adapting with medical advances, societal changes, regulatory constraints, consumer expectations, and other professional demands, the goal of the primary care provider (PCP) has remained to care for the patient as a person. Professional competencies and culture may vary between the primary care disciplines, yet all continue to emphasize health promotion in addition to the treatment of illness.[1–4] Indeed, despite the compelling forces of market competition, skewed payment systems, growing socioeconomic disparities, and a culture that increasingly

[a] Department of Family and Community medicine, SIU School of Medicine, 520 North 4th Street, Springfield, IL 62794-9670, USA; [b] Department of Family and Community medicine, SIU Center for Family Medicine, Quincy, IL, USA
* Corresponding author.
E-mail address: mdobbins@siumed.edu

Prim Care Clin Office Pract 43 (2016) 177–190
http://dx.doi.org/10.1016/j.pop.2016.01.003
0095-4543/16/$ – see front matter © 2016 Elsevier Inc. All rights reserved.
primarycare.theclinics.com

calls for convenience and expediency, primary care disciplines have protected the concept of holistic, patient-centered care in the setting of a medical home.[5]

The PCP not only possesses a vast array of medical skills and knowledge, but also continuously attempts to customize care in the context of the patient's individual personality and life circumstances, including family and community environment. Subsequently, PCPs have been called on to address increasingly complex issues, often coordinating a variety of limited resources and fragmented systems of care, while attempting to maintain patient engagement and satisfaction—all within the time constraints and fast pace of a busy medical practice.

Health Care Teams

Recognizing that these care demands are not always met by an individual provider, most practices have adopted a team approach to patient care. This is not a new concept, as physicians and nurses have traditionally worked together to provide care, and most practices have acquired a network of professionals to which they refer. Larger practices commonly designate staff teams that work together consistently to provide improved workflow and continuity of care. Team members may also review schedules or otherwise anticipate patient needs, enhancing efficiency and quality of care.

These examples share the commonality of arising out of adaptations to daily clinical practice, modifying the skills and duties of traditional professional staff. Over time, however, many practices have also begun to more formally and proactively structure care teams, assimilating groups of professionals whose composition reflects the needs of the patient population, practice interests of the providers, and availability (or scarcity) of local resources.

Multidisciplinary teams may come together in a variety of ways, proactively constructed, by gradual evolution, or even opportunistically through funding opportunities or organizational changes. They may develop methodically and intentionally with predetermined goals, evaluation processes, and proscribed timeline, or may evolve more slowly and subtly as practice personnel gradually recognize and are able to respond to emerging patient needs.[6]

The composition for one practice setting may not be desired or even feasible for another. Even within a practice setting, teams may change over time secondary to the availability of resources, priorities of leadership, evolution with practice need, or attrition and neglect. There are, however, certain characteristics of successful multidisciplinary teams (**Box 1**). With attention to such details, medical practice remains flexible and responsive to changes in patient care needs.[6–8]

Box 1
Characteristics of successful teams

Shared vision

Well-defined goals and expectations

Strong yet receptive leadership

Appropriate support structures

Well-defined roles

Inter-professional respect

Clear and frequent communication

Intermittent self-evaluation

Adaptability

Team Composition

Traditional disciplines have evolved and new health care professions have emerged in response to a burgeoning need for health care services in an environment of limited financial resources. Many health care disciplines have developed formal subcategories of credentials, with various educational requirements and professional competencies. Subsequently, even "primary care teams" may be quite diverse, having evolved to include an array of medical professionals who, depending on licensure, payer source, and local regulations, work with varying degrees of collaboration, supervision, or independence (**Box 2**).

Box 2 **Primary care teams**
Physicians (MD and DO)
Advance practice nurses (APN)
Physician assistants
Nurses (registered, licensed practical)
Certified nursing assistants
Certified medical assistants

The role of the office nurse has been especially pivotal, offering the professional flexibility to adapt to a variety of practice needs and provide expertise in a number of specialized areas (**Box 3**). As resources allow, many primary care practices also recruit professionals credentialed traditionally in other disciplines (**Box 4**), whose "colocated" practice may remain fairly traditional, well-defined, and self-sustaining, and whose value is readily understood and accepted by both patients and practice staff.

Box 3 **Diversity in nursing roles**
Direct primary care practice (APN)
General clinical assistance
Procedures
Screening
Education
Counseling
Case management
Administration
Research

Box 4 **"Colocated" services**
Pharmacists
Dieticians
Lactation consultants

As the medical needs and systems of care become more complex, however, many practices have also created new positions (**Box 5**) that greatly expand the concept of patient care by working between agencies, coordinating services, and tracking resource use and health outcomes. Unlike the former positions, these may have more fluid definitions and boundaries, be funded in a number of creative ways, and be filled by professionals with a variety of educational backgrounds. Indeed, the success of these positions is often highly dependent on the individual's interpersonal skills, which facilitate patient engagement and the development of collaborative professional partnerships.

Box 5
"Interdisciplinary" professionals

Case manager

Care coordinator

Patient navigator

Often, the holistic and patient-centered approach to care uncovers needs more social or environmental in nature. These may be best addressed by recruiting team members that would not necessarily be considered to be "medical" professionals (**Box 6**). When expanding into other disciplines, team members may work on a part-time or contractual basis if it is not feasible for them to function as full-time practice employees. In fact, anyone who has direct contact with patients (**Box 7**) may become very important in patient engagement, satisfaction, and medical care, functionally becoming part of the care team even if in a more informal fashion. The most important member of the "team," however, may be the recipient of care, the patient.

Box 6
"Nonmedical" professionals

Social workers

Legal consultants

Patient advocates

Educators

Box 7
Informal team members

Scribes

Receptionists

Referral specialists

Billing personnel

Telephone nurses

Peer counselors

Interpreters

Custodians

Security staff

BEHAVIORAL HEALTH
Components of Behavioral Health

Primary care disciplines have long recognized ways in which the patient contributes to their own health and health care. An almost endless number of individual factors (**Box 8**) vary greatly from person to person. These factors, often not obviously apparent, fully considered, or truly understood by the professional, motivate patient actions and may potentially promote or compromise health and treatment, be affected by health-related concerns, or affect resiliency and adjustment to everyday stressors.

As the medical profession has begun to recognize the importance of lifestyle, habits, and self-care, more professional efforts have been undertaken to influence patient health-related behaviors, leading to the development of an approach to care commonly referred to as "behavioral health."

Behavioral health is not a new concept; it has always been a part of primary care practice in some form, whether or not obviously recognized as such. In a more paternalistic era, it may have been somewhat concrete and prescriptive, telling a patient "what to do" to treat an illness, when to call, or when to present back to the office—all actionable behaviors on the part of the patient. Over time, however, a broader concept of behavioral health has become widely incorporated into the self-care emphasis of prenatal and health maintenance visits, and more targeted and formalized

---

Box 8
Personal characteristics

Personality

Cognitive skills

Executive function

General abilities

Resources

Education

Communication skills

Motivation

Habits

Interpersonal skills

Relationships

Life experiences

Spirituality

Cultural background

Trust

Bias

Expectations

Preferences

Fears

Coping skills

Self-regulation

programming is becoming more common for some adjustment problems, chronic illness, pain management, addictions, and mental health issues (**Box 9**).

Behavioral health = Engagement, Education, Motivation, Support

---

Whether formalized or not, all primary care practices provide some degree of behavioral health care, using a variety of models ranging from the use of written materials to individual appointments or group classes for education and support. The most effective behavioral health, however, expands on instruction and education to emphasize the importance of patient engagement, motivation, and support.[9–12]

Expansion of the Primary Care Team

Commonly, behavioral health services have been provided by the PCP, staff nurse or dietician, who does not necessarily require additional subspecialty training. Research in behavioral change, however, has also led to the inclusion of mental health professionals, who:

- Are adept at behavioral change techniques (motivational interviewing, supportive and cognitive-behavioral therapy, mindfulness and relaxation exercises)
- Facilitate patient engagement
- Explore the forces driving the behavior
- Recognize the need for more intensive mental health care
- Are familiar with a variety of additional resources

This has been especially helpful as PCPs, who have always recognized the interplay between mental and physical health, have begun to routinely use screening measures for substance abuse and mental health disorders. Secondarily, the inclusion of professionals trained in "mental health" has broadened both the breadth and depth of "behavioral health" (**Fig. 1**).

Programmatic Gaps

The practice of behavioral health has grown out of attempts to meet patient needs within the medical home. This development has been quite beneficial, as it has been customized per setting, and has also led to a more nuanced study of factors that affect health and quality of life. However, the development of behavioral health has also exposed gaps in traditional training models, as it has been considered to be an emerging type of care rather than a professional specialty. "Medical" professionals may struggle with the mental health aspects, and "mental health" providers may be unfamiliar with many aspects of medical illness, preventive care, and health maintenance. Many rely on some degree of cross-training.

From a practical point of view, the term "behavioral health" can cover a large variety of meanings and services, and may be used differently by professionals in different

---

Box 9
Areas of behavioral health

Self-care: safety, sleep, diet, weight management, exercise, general self-care

Adjustment Problems: grief, divorce

Chronic illness: obesity, diabetes, asthma, hypertension, pain management, addictions, mental illness

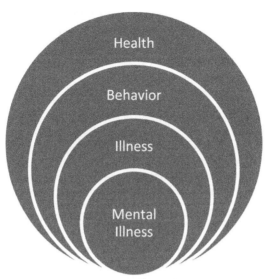

Fig. 1. Behavioral health/mental health spectrum. Behavioral health practices span from wellness to pathology, enhancing health and decreasing illness. Traditional mental health specialty care may be needed for a small percentage of a patient population.

settings. Likewise, the providers of behavioral health services may be known by a variety of titles and may have quite varied professional backgrounds, training, and credentials. Because this is such an important aspect of health care, however, programming continues to develop very quickly, with attempts to define "best practice" models for care and professional training that will promote integration of this type of patient care—paradoxically holistic yet "in between" traditional health care professions—into the medical home.

INTEGRATED CARE
Components of Integrated Care

Programmatic applications of these considerations have led to the concept of what is commonly called "integrated care." Historically considered from the perspective of the mental health disciplines, this is probably best described as the practice of using a mental health professional, typically a therapist (**Box 10**), within the medical setting and specifically emphasizes expansion of their service outside of colocated yet

---

Box 10
Integrated mental health professionals

Licensed clinical professional counselor (LCPC)

Licensed clinical social worker (LCSW)

Psychologist

Addiction specialist

Marriage and family counselor

Psychiatrist

traditional practice.[13,14] The integrated therapist may practice within the range of behavioral health concerns, but will also provide an additional expertise regarding mental health and substance abuse issues. As in medical practice, models and infrastructure may be quite varied; and the term does not indicate a standardized program. Conversely, however, "reverse integration" refers to the practice of using a medical professional within a mental health setting and typically consists of more traditional colocated services.[15–17]

Although a variety of professionals may provide this service, there are essential skill sets shared between all (**Box 11**). Customization is especially important, as emphasizing a colocated traditional model of the 1-hour therapy appointment will preclude the true integration of an expanded variety of clinical services, limit efforts at patient engagement, limit the number of patients assisted, and functionally isolate the therapist, stifling their ability to truly function as a member of the clinical treatment team.

Certainly, depending on available community resources and patient needs, some more traditional therapy visits may be provided, but should be considered as only a limited aspect of the therapist's role. The therapist who has experience with integrated care is, in fact, expanding the expertise of the discipline. In this context, being used for colocated traditional services, while technically allowing them to work at the top of their degree, is not functionally allowing them to work to the top of their ability, potentially wasting a valuable resource.

Clinical Aspects of Integrated Care

Clinical encounters will vary in duration, address a variety of issues, and use a variety of service techniques (**Box 12**). Because services will reflect the needs of the practice and, to some extent, the expertise and interests of the therapist, these may vary a great deal between settings. The employment of additional therapists is expected to expand types of services and flexibility in the provision of care, especially if team members coordinate their efforts. The common expectation, however, is for the therapist to create a visible presence in the clinical environment, readily available to be introduced to patients as they present for their primary care appointments, and easily accessed as a general resource for clinic staff.

The effective integrated therapist, while respecting the time constraints and professional boundaries of the clinical practice, will seek out contact with clinic staff members to develop familiarity and trust, encourage questions, and discuss services. This is not just a team-building role, but also assists in the ongoing assessment of clinical needs.

The ability to meet with a patient in need at the time of their medical appointment greatly facilitates patient engagement and follow-through with treatment recommendations, efficiency of clinic flow, and support of the medical staff.[14] To anticipate the need for assistance and plan accordingly for time and materials, many therapists

---

Box 11
Essential skills in behavioral health

Work with a variety of medical professionals with individual personalities in a fast-paced often high-stress setting

Quickly assess the needs of both the patient and the provider caring for the patient

Problem solve to provide a variety of interventions

Provide services in an adaptable, customized fashion

Box 12
Types of behavioral health assistance

Preclinic planning (huddles, schedule/chart review)

Provision of information, materials, resources

Patient deescalation

Assessment (brief or in depth)

Problem solving

Psychoeducation

Patient engagement

Linkage with additional care/services

Psychotherapy

Communication/coordination of care

Assessment of clinical needs

Program planning

---

routinely review the patients scheduled for the day, participate in preclinic "huddles," and otherwise routinely check in with clinic staff. However, the need for the therapist is frequently not anticipated until the provider is in the room with the patient. Subsequently, availability and responsiveness are of great importance.

The therapist may assist clinical staff by providing materials, suggesting resources, or otherwise answering questions, but typically will meet with the patient at the time of presentation, preferably introduced directly by the provider as a part of the clinical team. They may work in concert with the provider or complete the visit as the provider moves on with their schedule.

The encounter may be acute, as in the deescalation and in-depth assessment of a distraught patient. More commonly, however, it consists of psychoeducation, brief assessment and problem solving, or possibly just an introduction to facilitate engagement or schedule an appointment with the therapist.

Depending on clinic resources, scheduled visits with the therapist are usually arranged with the understanding that they may be interrupted if there is an acute clinic need. For certain patients, the therapist may suggest more intensive mental health services, including psychiatric care, and assist the provider in this referral process. If the therapist becomes aware of a medical concern during the course of their work with a patient, they facilitate communication with the referring provider to arrange further management.

Once a working relationship is established and services are well-understood, the provider may at times directly refer patients to the therapist without the intermediate step of the clinical introduction. However, caution should be taken not to jeopardize patient engagement, misuse the therapist as a resource, or overbook appointments at the expense of informal clinic availability (the main value of integrated care).

After an encounter, the therapist communicates with the provider to review outcomes and ongoing treatment planning. This may be done acutely if indicated, but oftentimes occurs in the form of brief weekly meetings or electronic communication. If the latter is used, consideration should be given regarding patient confidentiality and whether permanency within the medical record is desired. The therapist is always expected to provide routine documentation for any direct patient service.

The skills of the therapist are also easily applied as a practice consultant, who often can facilitate the patient experience and clinic flow, detect practice gaps, and develop programming to enhance employee health and decrease provider burnout.

The Role of the Psychiatrist

Psychiatrists may also provide services in the primary care setting, typically arranged as variations of colocated traditional practice. This arrangement can be especially helpful if intensive supportive services, a critical aspect of care for more severely ill psychiatric patients, are not needed or can be otherwise arranged.

Although typically more narrow in scope than the broad spectrum of behavioral health services provided by the integrated therapist, psychiatric care may also consist of a spectrum of services, including diagnostic evaluations, consultation sans direct treatment, and variations of limited medication management. Coverage and support issues typically preclude full ongoing psychiatric services within the primary care setting, however.

The availability of psychiatric treatment within the medical home decreases stigma, enhances patient engagement, and facilitates care.[16,18,19] In addition, the psychiatrist can assist in the determination of and facilitation for those who may need to be referred elsewhere for more intensive care. This is an important contribution to the cost-effective use of limited specialty resources, and has the added benefit of streamlining waiting time for the more severely ill. The psychiatrist who works closely with the integrated therapist can also develop a synergy and enhanced efficiency in the provision of patient care.

Similar to the integrated therapist, there are many ways in which a psychiatrist may expand their assistance in the practice. Having a presence in the clinic fosters better communication, understanding of the specialty, participation in comanagement and opportunities to function as an informal resource. In addition to patient care, the psychiatrist who provides liaison expertise can explore practice gaps, educational needs and population trends, and otherwise provide staff and program support. In general, the psychiatrist may provide psychiatric clinical services, but also provides psychiatric expertise to assist the PCPs in the care of their patients.

SYSTEMIC ASPECTS OF INTEGRATED CARE
Logistics

Most integrated care results in billable services, especially because there are a variety of additional codes that may be useful once there is an expansion upon traditional care (**Box 13**).[13,14] Even when certain services may not be directly billable, they provide

---

Box 13
Billing considerations

Variety of psychotherapy codes based on duration

Screening codes

Education codes

Complexity of interview

Crisis intervention

Group therapy

Coordination of services

value to patient care and may indirectly be contributing financially to the practice through enhanced provider efficiency. Most practices find it helpful to anticipate the amount of billing necessary to ensure the services of the therapist will be sustainable financially. It is of note that a therapist, who has a scheduled patient "no-show," may recoup that billing loss through the ability to participate in an unscheduled clinical encounter.

Planning should take into consideration special needs for space (especially for group sessions), staff support, supplies (especially for pediatric patients), screening tools, and brochures and printed materials as desired.

In addition to direct patient care, there are many systemic benefits to an integrated care approach. The introduction of integrated care complements case management and provides unique opportunities to track service use and outcomes at both the individual and population levels. Trends may emerge that indicate more targeted approaches to service in areas such as substance abuse, chronic pain management, diabetes/weight management, perinatal support, geriatric care, and developmental disabilities. Common contributing factors such as lack of transportation or food/housing insecurity may be identified. New practice-wide initiatives may be undertaken more effectively.

Stigma and Discomfort

In contrast with other practice innovations, integrating behavioral and mental health services may be significantly more vulnerable to the culture and attitude of office staff members at the individual level. Outdated yet pervasive stereotypes persist, and patients may be perceived as frightening, lazy, frustrating, or unworthy. Stigma may extend to the specialists and professional disciplines as well.[7] Additionally, mental health disciplines are often less familiar than other specialties, emergent symptoms are often ill-defined, services are poorly understood, and guidance for referral is often lacking. PCPs may fear "labeling" rather than "diagnosing" a patient, avoid potentially sensitive discussions, or feel awkward introducing the therapist and their services.

Communication and Language

Good communication is a challenge in any busy practice, especially in subjects historically treated with increased confidentiality. In addition, attempts to provide language for new concepts may have very different meanings to those with different backgrounds. For example, "warm hand-off," a phrase commonly used to refer to an in-person introduction, may be poorly accepted by those with a background of trauma or neglect. "Behaviorist," a term for the professional providing behavioral health services, may be rejected by those for whom it implies judgment or control.

Administration

The integrated professional constantly assesses clinical needs and responds in a fashion that is defining a new discipline, in essence adding the next layer to patient-centered care. However, administrative decisions are commonly based on traditional services in a "top-down" approach. Consideration should be given to compromise at the interface of the 2 approaches.[8]

OUTCOMES AND IMPLICATIONS
Clinical Care

Despite the lack of standardization or identity as a defined professional discipline, the integration of behavioral health care into the primary care setting has consistently demonstrated beneficial outcomes (**Box 14**). Patients remain more engaged, increase

---

Box 14
Outcomes of behavioral health care

Increased access to services

Increased patient engagement

Increased follow-through with treatment planning

Better response to care

Decreased stigma

Improved efficiency of care

Decreased overuse

Cost containment

Increased patient satisfaction

Increased provider satisfaction

---

their follow through with treatment plans, and have better response to care.[7,15,18,19] At the population level, this alleviates stigma, increases access to mental health services, enhances efficiency of care, decreases overuse of resources, and contains cost. Excessive primary care use is decreased, and education and support are systematized for the PCPs. In fact, this is a model of care that demonstrates increased satisfaction for both patients and providers.[7]

Medical Education

Although typically pursued for clinical reasons, integrated care provides significant educational opportunities for primary care staff through ongoing informal and formalized avenues. Discussion regarding both "what" is helpful and "why" quickly generalizes to systemized practice change. PCPs indicate a desire to learn more in regard to mental health care.[20,21] As practice gaps are identified, more structured programming can be provided through a variety of mechanisms, including staff meetings, quality assurance projects, or formalized continuing medical education offerings. In academic settings, where a designated curriculum may be instituted, this potential is profound. In fact, the Accreditation Council for Graduate Medical Education has formally recognized the need for training in behavioral/mental health in primary care programs.[22]

The implications for the education of mental health providers are equally as important, and new programming is beginning to address the concepts and skills necessary for this expanded type of practice.[6,8,17,20,21] Indeed, integrated clinics provide a unique opportunity for blended interdisciplinary educational efforts. Lessons learned from integrated care are especially expected to transform the practice of psychiatry. Not only will psychiatrists continue to improve the management of their patients' associated medical concerns, but for the first time have real opportunity to study the emergence of disorders in the clinical setting and explore the realm of preventative medicine—an approach of "primary care psychiatry."

Health Care Policy

Systems of care, professional training and licensure, funding mechanisms, and health policy have evolved over the years in a fashion that fails to adequately reduce disease and economic burden. However, new discoveries in neuroscience, epigenetics, trauma-informed care/toxic stress, and population health may truly be the "missing link," demonstrating how environment and life experiences physically contribute to the development of (and therefore the management of) chronic disease.[23,24] Integrated care is poised to meet this need and to transform both health care and health care policy, built on the solid foundation of the patient-centered medical home.

REFERENCES

1. American Academy of Family Physicians. Available at: www.aafp.org. Accessed August 1, 2015.
2. American Academy of Pediatrics. Available at: www.aap.org. Accessed August 1, 2015.
3. American College of Physicians. Available at: www.acponline.org. Accessed August 1, 2015.
4. American Congress of Obstetricians and Gynecologists. Available at: www.acog.org. Accessed August 1, 2015.
5. Phillips RI, Pugno PA, Saultz JW, et al. Health is primary: family medicine for America's health. Ann Fam Med 2014;12(Suppl 1):S1–12.
6. Adams T, Orchard C, Houghton P, et al. The metamorphosis of a collaborative team: from creation to operation. J Interprof Care 2014;28(4):339–44.
7. Brawer P, Martielli R, Pye P, et al. St. Louis initiative for integrated care excellence (SLI^{2}CE): integrated-collaborative care on a large scale model. Fam Syst Health 2010;28(2):175.
8. Hern T, Burke Valeras A, Banker J, et al. Collaborative partnerships within integrated behavioral health and primary care. In: Talen M, Burke Valeras A, editors. Integrated behavioral health in primary care. New York: Springer; 2013. p. 209–27.
9. Marvel MK, Doherty WJ, Weiner E. Medical interviewing by exemplary family physicians. J Fam Pract 1998;47(5):343–8.
10. Mauksch LB, Dugdale DC, Dodson S, et al. Relationship, communication and efficiency in the patient encounter: creating a clinical model from a literature review. Arch Intern Med 2008;168(13):1387–95.
11. Fischetti LR, McCutchan FC. A contextual history of the behavioral sciences in family medicine revisited. Fam Syst Health 2002;20:113–29.
12. Oyama O, Kosch SG, Burg MA, et al. Understanding the scope and practice of behavioral medicine in family medicine. Fam Med 2009;41(8):578–84.
13. Substance Abuse and Mental Health Services Administration. Available at: www.Integration.SAMSHA.gov. Accessed March 3, 2015.
14. National Council on Behavioral Health. Available at: www.thenationalcouncil.org. Accessed March 1, 2015.
15. Ratzliff A, Christensen C, Unützer J. Building value-added teams to care for behavioral health needs in primary care. In: Summergrad P, Kathol R, editors. Integrated care in psychiatry. New York: Springer; 2014. p. 103–26.
16. Barth FD. Building and working with an integrative team. In: Barth FD, editor. Integrative clinical social work practice. New York: Springer; 2014. p. 119–30.
17. Ivbijaro G, Enum Y, Khan A, et al. Collaborative care: models for treatment of patients with complex medical-psychiatric conditions. Curr Psychiatry Rep 2014; 16(11):1–12.
18. Oldham R, Hersevoort S. Integrated care: a population-based approach to consultation-liaison psychiatry. In: Leigh H, Strelzer J, editors. Handbook of consultation-liaison psychiatry. New York: Springer International Publishing; 2015. p. 115–28.

19. Unützer J, Katon W, Callahan C, et al. Collaborative-care management of late-life depression in the primary care setting. JAMA 2002;288(22):2836–45.
20. Thomas S, Dobbins M, Hill-Jordan J, et al. An investigation of primary care physicians attitudes toward psychiatry. Acad Psychiatry, in press.
21. Dobbins M, Roberts N, Vicari S, et al. The consultation conference: a mew model of collaboration for child psychiatry and primary care. Acad Psychiatry 2011; 35(4):260–2.
22. Accreditation Council for Graduate Medical Education. Available at: www.acgme. org. Accessed March 1, 2015.
23. Felitti VJ, Anda RF, Nordenberg D, et al. Relationship of childhood abuse and household dysfunction to many of the leading causes of death in adults. The Adverse Childhood Experiences (ACE) Study. Am J Prev Med 1998;14(4): 245–58.
24. Garner A, Shonkoff J, the Committee on Psychosocial Aspects of Child and Family Health (Siegel B, Dobbins M, Earls M, McGuinn L, Pascoe J, and Wood D). Policy statement- early childhood adversity, toxic stress, and the role of the pediatrician: translating developmental science into lifelong health. Pediatrics 2012; 129(1):e224–31. Elk Grove Village, IL. The American Academy of Pediatrics.

Behavioral Health in Prevention and Chronic Illness Management
Motivational Interviewing

Donna Tuccero, MD, Kenyon Railey, MD,
Melvania Briggs, MA, PA-C, Sharon K. Hull, MD, MPH*

KEYWORDS

- Motivational interviewing • Prevention • Behavior change • Chronic illness
- Primary care • Collaborative care

KEY POINTS

- Health outcomes, including chronic illness morbidity and mortality, are directly influenced by patient choices.
- Motivational interviewing (MI) techniques were originally developed to address substance abuse disorders but are now being used to address the primary and secondary prevention of a variety of health behaviors and chronic illnesses.
- MI is a tool clinicians can use to actively engage patients in their care.
- The spirit of MI, as described by the creators of MI, is based on collaboration, compassion, evocation, and patient autonomy with an emphasis on empathy and empowerment.

INTRODUCTION

Motivational interviewing (MI) was developed approximately 30 years ago by psychologist William R. Miller, PhD as a tool for evoking behavior change, primarily for use with clients in addressing substance abuse.[1] It has been widely used and validated as effective in this setting. Its usefulness has also spread to a variety of conditions unrelated to substance abuse. The purpose of this article is to address the effectiveness of MI in prevention of illness and in management of long-term chronic disease, with an emphasis on its use in primary care.

Disclosure Statement: The authors have no financial or other substantive conflicts of interest to disclose.
Department of Community and Family Medicine, Duke University School of Medicine, 2100 Erwin Road, Durham, NC 27710, USA
* Corresponding author.
E-mail address: sharon.hull@duke.edu

Prim Care Clin Office Pract 43 (2016) 191–202
http://dx.doi.org/10.1016/j.pop.2016.01.006   primarycare.theclinics.com
0095-4543/16/$ – see front matter © 2016 Elsevier Inc. All rights reserved.

DEFINITION

MI was originally described in 1983 as "a patient communication style that utilizes guidance and goal directing in order to elicit and emphasize individual motivations for change."[1] A comprehensive theoretic model for MI has been developed and refined over time.[2] Rollnick and Miller[3] defined MI as "a directive, client-centered counseling style for eliciting behavior change by helping clients to explore and resolve ambivalence."[3] In 2009, the creators of MI offered an updated definition stating "Motivational Interviewing is a collaborative, person-centered form of guiding to elicit and strengthen motivation for change."[4] The spirit of MI arises from the assumption of collaborative partnership, acceptance of the client's autonomy and perspective, compassion (keeping the client's best interests in mind), and evocation (an understanding that "the best ideas come from the client").[5,6]

The focus of the method is based on a set of skills often referred to as OARS: asking open questions; providing affirmations of patients' positive behaviors, beliefs, and accomplishments; reflective listening; and summary statements.[5,7] **Box 1** describes key principles guiding the implementation of MI. Comprehensive formal training in MI can be obtained online or in person from a variety of sources, including a framework and curriculum for training resident physicians in family medicine and psychiatry[8] as well as other prescribing providers (nurse practitioners and physician assistants).[9]

IMPORTANCE OF THE TOPIC: SCOPE

With the advent of cutting-edge biomedical technologies and the advancement of evidence-based medicine during the past century, the ability to diagnose and respond to life-threatening illness has positively contributed to the prolongation of life and prevention of long-term morbidity. In spite of the historic advances, the current health care system is not designed to support prevention or to reduce the progression of chronic illness.[10]

Most deaths among individuals in the United States are related to chronic illnesses. such as heart disease, cerebrovascular disease, diabetes, and certain cancers. These conditions are, simultaneously, common and costly for individuals and institutions. In 2012, nearly 50% of adult Americans had at least one chronic illness and approximately 26% of adults had multiple chronic illnesses.[11] Analysis has shown that nearly

---

Box 1
Capturing the spirit of motivational interviewing

1. Motivation to change is elicited from the patients, not imposed from outside.
2. It is the patients' task, not the physician's, to resolve their ambivalence.
3. Direct persuasion is not an effective method for resolving ambivalence.
4. The counseling style is a quiet one, with a focus on eliciting the patients' thoughts.
5. The physician is directive in helping patients examine and resolve ambivalence.
6. Readiness to change is not a patient trait but a fluctuating product of interpersonal interaction.
7. The therapeutic relationship is more like a partnership or companionship; expert/recipient roles can impede the process.

For more information, visit http://www.motivationalinterview.net.
From Stewart EE, Fox CH. Encouraging patients to change unhealthy behaviors with motivational interviewing. Fam Pract Manag 2011;18(3):21–5.

half of all deaths in the United States can be attributed to preventable causes.[12,13] (**Table 1** presents a summary of this data.) This recent analysis focuses on upstream preventable causes of death rather than death certificate reports.

Health outcomes, chronic illness morbidity, and mortality are all directly influenced by choices that patients make. Of the 10 health indicators identified in the Healthy People 2010 initiative, 5 were directly related to personal health behaviors.[14] Healthy People 2020 builds on the 2010 report but adds 2 additional objectives, one of which involves the promotion of healthy behaviors across life stages.[15]

Clinician knowledge and communication remain at the cornerstone of patient care, yet health care providers of all types truly have little direct command over patient behavior choices (ie, smoking cessation, participation in regular exercise, medication, and diet adherence) that contribute to optimum health and avoidance of chronic illness. Absence of control, however, does not imply absence of influence, as this article demonstrates.

Behavior change is also at the core of patient care, which provides the foundation of intervention through prevention. Ultimately, although prevention efforts at various levels are paramount, achieving behavior change depends on patients' ability to modify harmful behavior and institute healthy behavioral substitutes. Preventive medicine interventions are classically described within 3 categories. **Table 2** presents these definitions and examples of specific prevention interventions for each.

To truly influence behavior change, tools have been developed to assist patients with making more healthful and helpful choices. MI is one such technique. It creates opportunities to influence patients' choices by helping them manage their ambivalence about behavior change and self-identify barriers and successes.[5]

SUPPORTING EVIDENCE

The chronic care model[16–19] was developed in part as a response to understanding of the limitations of the current health care delivery system in addressing chronic disease. One of its core elements is support of self-management, which emphasizes

Table 1	
Actual causes of death, United States, 2000	
Actual Cause of Death	**Percent of all Deaths in the United States (2000)**
Tobacco use	18.1
Poor diet and physical inactivity	16.6
Alcohol consumption	3.5
Microbial agents	3.1
Toxic agents	2.3
Motor vehicle	1.8
Firearms	1.2
Sexual behavior	0.8
Illicit drug use	0.7
Total deaths (percent of all deaths) from these causes	1,159,000 (48.2)

Data from Mokdad AH, Marks JS, Stroup DF, et al. Actual causes of death in the United States, 2000. JAMA 2004;291(10):1238–45; and Mokdad AH, Marks JS, Stroup DF, et al. Correction: actual causes of death in the United States, 2000. JAMA 2005;293(3):293–4.

Table 2
Levels of prevention

	Definition	Examples
Primary prevention	Focuses on individuals who do not yet have a disease and provides interventions that are aimed at reducing the likelihood that they will develop a disease	Immunization and promotion of physical activity and healthy dietary choices
Secondary prevention	Focuses on individuals who have a disease but who are not yet symptomatic and aims to detect and manage this presymptomatic disease	Screening for cancer, hyperlipidemia, hypertension, and diabetes in patients who have not already been diagnosed with the condition being screened
Tertiary prevention	Focuses on individuals who have a disease and are symptomatic from that disease, aiming to limit the progression of that disease to include disability or premature death	Most care of acute and chronic illness by physicians as well as rehabilitation services

Adapted from Katz DL, Ali A. Preventive medicine, integrative medicine and the health of the public. Washington, DC: Institute of Medicine; 2009.

individual and group efforts to maximize patient empowerment.[20] This element of chronic disease care and management is likely most amenable to the use of MI techniques.

MI arose from the mental health arena, specifically as it related to addiction treatment; thus, many reviews of MI efficacy have examined studies conducted outside traditional primary care settings. With the current emphasis on chronic disease management in primary care and the recognition of need for patient investment in their care, MI has been increasingly either piloted or embedded in existing programs in primary care medicine, across a wide range of conditions and related behaviors.

Obesity

Given the overall increase in obesity rates both nationally[21] and internationally,[22] it is not surprising that several studies have focused on the role of MI in weight loss as primary prevention in at-risk populations. A systematic review of 11 randomized controlled trials (RCTs) conducted from 1995 to 2009 investigated the effectiveness of MI for reducing body mass in patients with hypertension, diabetes type 2, hyperlipidemia, inactivity, or job-related risk. End points included change in body weight or body mass index (BMI) in overweight or obese adults.[23] Delivery of MI was performed by interviewers from diverse professional backgrounds. Intervention varied both by intervention type (individual, group, and telephone sessions) and duration as calculated by the number of sessions and duration. The weighted mean decrease of 1.47 kg of body weight in the intervention arm was statistically significant. The greatest amount of weight loss was associated with duration of MI longer than 6 months, interviewer fidelity, and combining MI with a group-based behavioral weight loss program. MI seemed to increase attendance by participants at the behavioral program, thus, resulting in improved adherence.

Physical Activity

In addition to maintenance of healthy body weight, regular moderate-intensity physical activity is recommended for patients to decrease the risk of chronic health conditions, including cardiovascular disease.[24] A 2014 systematic review and meta-analysis from Australia assessed the effectiveness of MI on increasing physical activity in people with chronic health conditions, including obesity, hypertension, hyperlipidemia, peripheral arterial disease, multiple sclerosis, fibromyalgia, and coronary artery disease.[25] Ten RCTs were included and represented not only primary care clinics but also community health centers or community residential sites. MI had a small but significant effect on increasing physical activity in this study. Adherence to MI treatment fidelity led to improved efficacy of the intervention, although there was no evidence that mode of delivery impacted outcomes.

Treatment Engagement

MI has been used in various scenarios to promote treatment adherence. Most studies focused on medication adherence or the extent to which patients' history of therapeutic drug taking coincides with the prescribed treatment. This issue is a particular problem in the elderly who are more likely to have multiple chronic diseases and, thereby, take multiple medications. An RCT conducted in 16 primary care health centers in Spain assessed medication adherence in elderly patients who were taking more than 5 medications.[26] Individualized MI was provided as part of the visit by their provider or nurse. At the end of the treatment period, participants in the MI group increased their treatment adherence 24.3% versus 16.7% for those in the control group.

Delivery methods for MI vary across studies, and there are mixed results as to whether this significantly impacts outcomes. Some interventions have used only face-to-face interviews, whereas others have used group or telephone interventions. A review of 9 RCTs or cohort studies between 1990 and 2012 evaluated the effect of nontraditional MI delivery methods on medication adherence in patients with a variety of chronic illnesses.[27] The telephone was chosen as part of the medication adherence intervention because MI delivered by telephone had previously been shown effective for several end points. The premise of the study review was that providers have limited patient contact time in any given day and that other team members could provide the phone counseling. Underserved patients also have less access to reliable transportation, which limits opportunities for behavior education or change interventions; thus, the telephone could potentially impact this population. Adherence was determined by self-report and verified by pharmacy fills and insurance claims. Improved adherence was seen for patients with multiple sclerosis, mental illness, and coronary artery disease with comorbid diabetes mellitus. A cohort study showed a positive effect for medication adherence in osteoporosis and human immunodeficiency virus (HIV), but this was not supported by the RCT findings. Interestingly, subgroup analysis showed a positive effect on the 65- to 74-year-old osteoporotic group but not on those aged 75 years or older, suggesting differing responses to MI according to age group.

Chronic Pain

A community-based intervention of MI coupled with physical therapy for persons greater than 65 years of age with chronic pain was conducted in Hong Kong. End points included pain measures and quality of life. The combination of MI and physical exercise demonstrated improvements in pain intensity, pain self-efficacy, physical mobility, and psychological well-being.[28]

Diabetes Mellitus

The DYNAMIC (Diabetes nurse case management and motivational interviewing for change) trial was a 2-year RCT of 545 patients analyzing the effect of MI on parameters of diabetes control.[29] Although this RCT recruited patients from an endocrine outpatient clinic, the implications for primary care are relevant. Nurse case managers received an intense 80-hour training course in MI, and fidelity to MI approach was monitored. Both the control and intervention groups achieved equal reductions in hemoglobin A1c (HbA1c) (1.0% and 1.1%), low-density lipoprotein cholesterol, and diastolic blood pressure. Within the intervention group, a slight systolic blood pressure decrease and improved depression symptom scores were realized. Of note, most patients recruited were low income and 39% were Hispanic.

These results stand in contrast to a positive effect on HbA1c levels seen in a more homogenous patient population. In the 12-month diabetes management program known as the Happy Life Club,[30] diabetic patients older than 55 years were recruited in Beijing, China. The intervention group showed statistically significant improvements in HbA1c, but the clinical effect was quite small (mean change HbA1c of 0.4%). Improvements were likewise seen for systolic blood pressure and quality of life in the intervention group.

Systematic Review of Multiple Conditions in General Medical Settings

A variety of other end points have been studied in the primary care setting as well. Lundahl and colleagues,[31] in a large meta-analysis of 48 studies representing 9618 participants, evaluated MI within general medical care settings across a variety of chronic conditions. The goal of the study was to determine if MI was a potential treatment option within the delivery of routine medical care for these conditions. Locations of care were exceedingly diverse and included hospital clinics, medical outpatient clinics, the emergency department, women's health centers, weight loss clinics, and dental offices. Overall, MI showed a statistically significant beneficial effect in 63% of comparisons. Looking at disease or problem type, benefits were evident in 17 diverse parameters. **Table 3** summarizes the findings from this systematic review. The overall findings indicated that MI was effective in primary medical care settings as well as in previously proven addiction and medical specialty clinics.

Cultural Variability

Heterogeneity of study group composition may be impacting the MI effect as evidenced by subgroup analysis. For example, in Armstrong and colleagues'[23] systematic review of weight loss, 2 studies showed that MI failed to improve weight loss outcomes as compared with the control group of African American women. Witt and colleagues[32] cited these studies in a review in 2013, which analyzed the existing literature on the use of MI as a behavioral intervention to reduce cardiovascular disease risk among African American and Latina women. Only 7 published studies met the inclusion criteria for this systematic review. Overall, the MI results were inconsistent when applied to reducing cardiovascular risk factors in African American and Latina women. There were, however, statistically significant effects on increasing fruit and vegetable consumption across African American women. For the Latinas, MI showed positive trends in lowering SBP and achieving weight loss goals.

In an effort to provide culturally appropriate MI interventions, a multicenter MI trial addressing cancer risk factor reduction in Latinos[33] focused on a search for an adaptation to a traditional MI program. The goal was to identify models of cultural sensitivity and culturally appropriate educational materials in order to target the cluster of tobacco use, poor nutrition, and physical inactivity behaviors. Investigators used input from local focus groups to identify cultural values and assess pretest educational materials. A pilot test was performed in 2014, and a 400-patient study is planned for 2015.

Table 3
Effect of motivational interviewing in medical care settings

Outcomes	Positive Effect	Neutral Effect	Negative Effect
Biometrics	Blood pressure Cholesterol HIV viral load	Heart rate Blood glucose	—
Habits	Dangerous ETOH use Tobacco Marijuana	—	—
Risk reduction behaviors	Body weight BMI Waist circumference	Bicycle helmet use Riding with drunk driver Condom use No. of sexual partners Reporting STD status	Binge/purge behavior
Physical functioning & quality of life	Physical strength 6 Quality-of-life indicators in chronic disease (type 2 diabetes, stroke, and congestive heart failure)	Functional independence	—
Patient engagement with recommended therapeutic plans	Keeping appointments Participating in treatment plan Self-monitoring: glucose, food diary, physical activity Readiness to change	Epilepsy self-care Epilepsy medication Breast feeding	—
Disease end points	Dental caries Death	—	—

Abbreviations: ETOH, ethanol; STD, sexually transmitted disease.
Adapted from Lundahl B, Moleni T, Burke BL, et al. Motivational interviewing in medical care settings: a systematic review and meta-analysis of randomized controlled trials. Patient Educ Couns 2013;93(2):157–68.

Overall, MI shows promise for utilization in the primary care setting to activate patients and engage them in their health care. It has been used solely or in combination with other educational efforts and programs in a variety of chronic conditions. Statistically significant effects are generally positive, although often small. Subgroup analyses reveal that cultural adaptation of the technique to special populations is required if MI is to be of benefit in these groups.

APPLICATION

Use of MI in the primary care setting has many applications; but in order to deliver appropriate MI, practitioners need to couple the spirit of MI with a common set of skills. Within the spirit of MI, readiness to change is not seen as a patient trait but as a byproduct of patient-provider interaction. Motivation to change is evoked in patients rather than imposed.[3] When the techniques are applied, the provider can collaborate with patients to facilitate health-promoting behavior change and resolve any ambivalence. Its use is closely linked to helping patients move through the stages of change, which is a model developed by James Prochaska and Carlo DiClemente, and later refined by them and John Norcross[34] in the late 1970s. This theory posits that people go through a fairly predictable and autonomous process when making behavior change. Any useful treatment method must correspond to the individual's readiness to change. The spirit of MI emphasizes patient autonomy while drawing out individual thoughts about change rather than imposing provider ideas. **Fig. 1** describes the stages of change developed by Prochaska and DiClemente and includes examples of MI techniques in relationship to the model. **Fig. 1** directs the provider through each stage with a description of patient presentation, provider strategy and goal, and then an example of an MI technique to keep the process moving forward.

Box 1 (already referenced earlier) outlines core principles of effective MI. Key practical strategies and sample language for delivering effective MI in the clinical setting are found in **Table 4**. Other important issues include setting a clear agenda with patients, asking open-ended questions, practicing active listening when hearing the

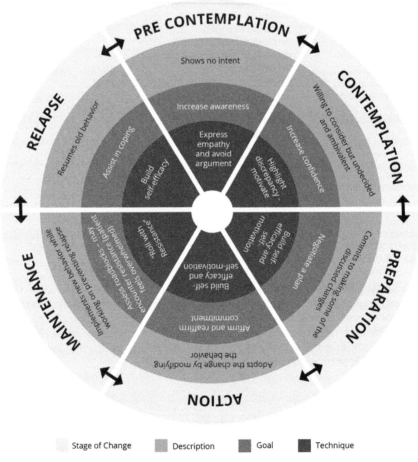

Fig. 1. Application of the stages of change. (*Adapted from* Prochaska JO, Di Clemente CC, Norcross JC. In search of how people change. Applications to addictive behaviors. Am Psychol 1992;47(9):1102–14; and Prochaska JO, Velicer WF. The transtheoretical model of health behavior change. Am J Health Promot 1997;12(1):38–48.)

Table 4
Practical application techniques for effective motivational interviewing

	Technique	Sample Language
1.	Express empathy and avoid arguments	I understand you have tried to stop smoking in the past and it has been hard. Many people find it difficult to stop smoking. I still think that it is important to your health. What are some things you think you could do to prepare to stop smoking?
2.	Highlight discrepancies in behavior	You have said that you would like to be able to move around with less pain. It seems like you know that exercise would help you achieve that goal. Why do you think it is hard for you to plan time for exercise?
3.	"Roll with resistance" using personalized feedback	I know you have a busy schedule, but do you think you could try planning for healthy meal preparation on one of your regular days off work, such as the weekend?
4.	Build self-efficacy and self-motivation	Let us talk about what you can do to reduce your intake of refined sugar.

From Motivational interviewing: a tool for behavior change. ACOG Committee Opinion No. 423. American College of Obstetricians and Gynecologists. Obstet Gynecol 2009;113:243–6; with permission.

patients' responses, helping patients to elicit their own understanding of the importance of the behavior change under consideration, and building and supporting confidence in the patients' ability to make the desired behavior change, described as enhancing self-efficacy.

PRACTICAL ISSUES

There are a few practical issues regarding the implementation of MI in primary care settings. Traditional medical training has not included principles of MI.[35] Silberberg and colleagues[36] surveyed providers at 13 primary care practices to assess perceptions regarding pediatric obesity treatment. The investigators found that primary care provider comfort and confidence were low for the ability to conduct MI. Because MI can be considered a paradigm shift for many providers and confidence can be low, practitioners not adequately trained in patient-centered counseling will likely require at least basic instruction in MI techniques.

The core skills and strategies of MI (eg, asking open-ended questions, agenda setting, reflective listening) are likely achievable in a few hours or days of training. Fu and colleagues,[37] however, suggested that more intensive instruction likely improves MI proficiency. In this study, the investigators evaluated outcomes of implementation of 2 training models for MI techniques for primary care providers to address tobacco abuse. In this study, 34 clinicians all received a single half-day workshop facilitated by MI expert trainers. Eighteen of the participants were randomly assigned to high-intensity training, which involved more training sessions, telephone interactions with simulated patients, and peer coaching over a 3-month period. A structured clinical evaluation 12 weeks after the initial training found that there were significant gains in proficiency in MI counseling knowledge, skills, and confidence in the high-intensity-training group.

The type and intensity of training will vary by provider and institutional interest, time, and availability. Despite the variability that exists in the literature regarding instructional methods, settings, and outcomes, most studies reveal gains in comfort and confidence after training. A successful MI training for primary care providers was instituted in the Veterans Health Administration, finding that "brief MI training protocols can lead to increased provider knowledge and confidence, and self-reported usage of MI skills in clinical practice."[9] Australia's Victorian Council on Physical Activity and General Health has outlined a practical how-to approach for general practitioners to use MI within a busy office setting for motivating patients to improve physical activity.[38] This approach can be applied to other clinical conditions as well.

Potential practitioners of MI may be reluctant to adapt or adopt interviewing or counseling techniques given the perception that time will be increased and reimbursement reduced. An MI study conducted to address weight loss prediction 3 months after an encounter concluded that patients whose providers used MI-consistent techniques achieved weight loss at 3 months after the encounter compared with patients whose providers did not. Encounters with patients who had a higher "Motivational Interviewing spirit score," a scale that contained 3 components of evocation, collaboration, and autonomy, were 61.9 seconds longer than those with lower spirit scores. Overall encounters were 63.4 seconds shorter when providers used behaviors consistent with accepted MI techniques.[39]

Although MI has broad applications in health promotion and disease prevention, it remains unclear how practitioners should be consistently compensated.[40] The shifting reimbursement environment and the planned implementation of new coding and billing techniques will have an impact on provider reimbursement, which cannot be fully predicted. Providers have historically been able to use traditional Evaluation and Management service codes for such reimbursement. In an environment increasingly driven by a patient-centered approach to creating value in health care, techniques such as MI may demonstrate value and, thus, continue to be reimbursable; this remains to be seen over time.

OUTCOMES

As is clear from the aforementioned evidence, there is support for the use of MI in improving biological markers, reducing risky habitual behaviors, improving physical functioning and quality of life, enhancing engagement with therapeutic plans, and reducing the prevalence of end points for some diseases, including mortality. It is unclear whether the lack of standardization of MI delivery impacted the variability of findings related to the effectiveness of MI interventions. Further study is needed to determine whether a uniform delivery style, in terms of frequency of contact or duration of intervention, would impact results.

SUMMARY/DISCUSSION

Usefulness of MI has grown beyond its origins in management of substance abuse, and it can be a beneficial tool for several conditions that are very common in primary care. Its use may require a philosophic shift in the patient-provider encounter for some practitioners. Its core principles of empathy, discrepancy development, adjustment for resistance, and self-efficacy support focus on change through patient-centered collaboration. MI is an active process that seeks to engage patients in the decision-making process toward behavior change.

Practitioners of MI come from a wide variety of disciplines, including psychologists, nurses, counselors, social workers, and medical providers. With proper training, primary care providers can learn to apply MI techniques to a wide array of health behaviors as they relate to chronic illness. Skillful practitioners can switch between various communication techniques, using MI as one of many tools, when appropriate, based on patient and provider needs.

REFERENCES

1. Miller WR. Motivational interviewing with problem drinkers. Behav Psychother 1983;11(2):147–72.
2. Miller WR, Rollnick S. Motivational interviewing: preparing people for change. New York: The Guilford Press; 2002.
3. Rollnick S, Miller WR. What is motivational interviewing? Behav Cogn Psychother 1995;23:325–34.
4. Miller WR, Rollnick S. Ten things that motivational interviewing is not. Behav Cogn Psychother 2009;37(2):129–40.
5. Matulich B. Introduction to motivational interviewing. YouTube; 2013. Available at: https://youtube/s3MCJZ7OGRk. Accessed March 8, 2016.
6. Rollnick S, Miller WR, Butler CC. Motivational interviewing in health care: helping patients change behavior. New York: The Guilford Press; 2008.
7. Stewart EE, Fox CH. Encouraging patients to change unhealthy behaviors with motivational interviewing. Fam Pract Manag 2011;18(3):21–5.
8. Triana AC, Olson MM, Trevino DB. A new paradigm for teaching behavior change: implications for residency training in family medicine and psychiatry. BMC Med Educ 2012;12:64.
9. Cucciare MA, Ketroser N, Wilbourne P, et al. Teaching motivational interviewing to primary care staff in the Veterans Health Administration. J Gen Intern Med 2012;27(8):953–61.
10. Benjamin RM. The national prevention strategy: shifting the nation's health-care system. Public Health Rep 2011;126(6):774–6.
11. Ward BW, Schiller JS, Goodman RA. Multiple chronic conditions among US adults: a 2012 update. Prev Chronic Dis 2014;11:E62.
12. Mokdad AH, Marks JS, Stroup DF, et al. Actual causes of death in the United States, 2000. JAMA 2004;291(10):1238–45.
13. Mokdad AH, Marks JS, Stroup DF, et al. Correction: actual causes of death in the United States, 2000. JAMA 2005;293(3):293–4.
14. Centers for Disease Control and Prevention. Healthy People 2010 leading health indicators at a glance. 2015. Available at: http://www.cdc.gov/nchs/healthy_people/hp2010/hp2010_indicators.htm.
15. Koh HK. A 2020 vision for healthy people. N Engl J Med 2010;362(18):1653–6.
16. Wagner EH. Chronic disease management: what will it take to improve care for chronic illness? Eff Clin Pract 1998;1(1):2–4.
17. Wagner EH, Austin BT, Davis C, et al. Improving chronic illness care: translating evidence into action. Health Aff 2001;20(6):64–78.
18. Wagner EH, Austin BT, Von Korff M. Organizing care for patients with chronic illness. Milbank Q 1996;74(4):511–44.
19. Wagner EH, Austin BT, Von Korff M. Improving outcomes in chronic illness. Manag Care Q 1996;4(2):12–25.
20. Liu G, Perkins A, Duffy L. Improving our approach to preventive care. J Fam Pract 2015;64(6):343–8.
21. Centers for Disease Control and Prevention. Adult obesity facts. 2015. Available at: http://www.cdc.gov/obesity/data/adult.html. Accessed July 29, 2015.
22. World Health Organization. Obesity and overweight: fact sheet. 2015. Available at: http://www.who.int/mediacentre/factsheets/fs311/en/. Accessed July 29, 2015.
23. Armstrong MJ, Mottershead TA, Ronksley PE, et al. Motivational interviewing to improve weight loss in overweight and/or obese patients: a systematic review and meta-analysis of randomized controlled trials. Obes Rev 2011;12(9):709–23.

24. National Institutes of Health. Physical activity guidelines for Americans. Washington, DC: National Institutes of Health; 2008.

25. O'Halloran PD, Blackstock F, Shields N, et al. Motivational interviewing to increase physical activity in people with chronic health conditions: a systematic review and meta-analysis. Clin Rehabil 2014;28(12):1159–71.

26. Moral RR, Torres LA, Ortega LP, et al. Effectiveness of motivational interviewing to improve therapeutic adherence in patients over 65 years old with chronic diseases: a cluster randomized clinical trial in primary care. Patient Educ Couns 2015;98(8):977–83.

27. Teeter BS, Kavookjian J. Telephone-based motivational interviewing for medication adherence: a systematic review. Transl Behav Med 2014;4(4):372–81.

28. Tse MM, Vong SK, Tang SK. Motivational interviewing and exercise programme for community-dwelling older persons with chronic pain: a randomised controlled study. J Clin Nurs 2013;22(13–14):1843–56.

29. Gabbay RA, Anel-Tiangco RM, Dellasega C, et al. Diabetes nurse case management and motivational interviewing for change (DYNAMIC): results of a 2-year randomized controlled pragmatic trial. J Diabetes 2013;5(3):349–57.

30. Browning CJ, Yang H, Zhang T, et al. Implementing a chronic disease self-management program into china: the happy life club. Front Public Health 2014; 2:181.

31. Lundahl B, Moleni T, Burke BL, et al. Motivational interviewing in medical care settings: a systematic review and meta-analysis of randomized controlled trials. Patient Educ Couns 2013;93(2):157–68.

32. Witt DR, Lindquist R, Treat-Jacobson D, et al. Motivational interviewing to reduce cardiovascular risk in African American and Latina women. West J Nurs Res 2013;35(10):1266–79.

33. Castro Y, Fernandez ME, Strong LL, et al. Adaptation of a counseling intervention to address multiple cancer risk factors among overweight/obese Latino smokers. Health Educ Behav 2015;42(1):65–72.

34. Prochaska JO, DiClemente CC, Norcross JC. In search of how people change. Applications to addictive behaviors. Am Psychol 1992;47(9):1102–14.

35. Committee on Health Care for Underserved Women. Motivational interviewing: a tool for behavior change. American College of Obstetrics and Gynecology; 2009. Available at: http://www.acog.org/Resources-And-Publications/Committee-Opinions/Committee-on-Health-Care-for-Underserved-Women/Motivational-Interviewing-A-Tool-for-Behavior-Change. Accessed March 8, 2016.

36. Silberberg M, Carter-Edwards L, Murphy G, et al. Treating pediatric obesity in the primary care setting to prevent chronic disease: perceptions and knowledge of providers and staff. N C Med J 2012;73(1):9–14.

37. Fu SS, Roth C, Battaglia CT, et al. Training primary care clinicians in motivational interviewing: a comparison of two models. Patient Educ Couns 2015;98(1):61–8.

38. Huang N. Motivating patients to move. Aust Fam Physician 2005;34(6):413–7.

39. Pollak KI, Alexander SC, Coffman CJ, et al. Physician communication techniques and weight loss in adults: project CHAT. Am J Prev Med 2010;39(4):321–8.

40. Resnicow K, Dilorio C, Soet JE, et al. Motivational interviewing in health promotion: it sounds like something is changing. Health Psychol 2002;21(5):444–51.

Using Cognitive Behavior Therapy and Mindfulness Techniques in the Management of Chronic Pain in Primary Care

CrossMark

Norah Baker, MD

KEYWORDS

- Chronic pain • Mental illness • Depression • Behavioral therapy • Mindfulness

KEY POINTS

- Chronic pain has become more prevalent than many common chronic illnesses, such as heart disease and diabetes, which has led to an increase in prescribing narcotic pain medications and subsequent increase in adverse events and mortality.
- Using advanced imaging modalities, it has been shown that depression and pain perception activate the same areas of the brain.
- Chronic pain syndrome occurs in patients who experience pain and disability for a longer period time than was reasonably expected.
- Depression and substance abuse are commonly seen concurrently with chronic pain and can be used as a red flag for poor outcome. The Patient Health Questionnaire and Alcohol Use Disorders Identification Test-C (AUDIT-C) are evidence-based screening tools for depression and substance abuse, respectively.
- Mindfulness techniques and cognitive behavior therapy can be used to help patients better manage their chronic pain and increase activity.

INTRODUCTION

Treating patients with chronic pain has become increasingly difficult for primary care physicians. In 2011, the Institute of Medicine (IOM) reported that pain affects an estimated 100 million Americans and has become more common than many chronic conditions, including diabetes, coronary heart disease, stroke, and cancer (**Table 1**).[1–3] At the same time, the number of prescriptions for pain medications has been increasing, as well as the number of subsequent deaths associated with overdose and drug interactions (**Fig. 1**). During this period of rapid growth in narcotic use, the prevalence of chronic pain has remained stable since 2006, forcing physicians to realize that the fault

---

Disclosures: The author has nothing to disclose, and has received no financial compensation for writing this article.
Red Bud Clinic Corporation, 415 West South 4th Street, Red Bud, IL 62278, USA
E-mail address: i.am.norahbakermd@gmail.com

Table 1
Incidence of chronic pain in the United States compared with other common chronic illnesses

Condition	Estimated Incidence in United States: 2011	Source of Data
Chronic pain	100 million	IOM
Diabetes	25.8 million (diagnosed and estimated less than-diagnosed)	ADA
Coronary heart disease (MI or angina)	16.3 million	AHA
Stroke	7 million	AHA
Cancer	11.9 million	ACS

Abbreviations: ACS, American Cancer Society; ADA, American Diabetes Association; AHA, American Health Association; MI, myocardial infarction.

Data from American Academy of Pain Medicine. AAPM facts and figures on pain. 2011. Available at: http://www.painmed.org/patientcenter/facts_on_pain.aspx#refer. Accessed July 6, 2015.

lies with overprescribing of pain medications, with guidelines for appropriate treatment and monitoring newly prioritized.[4]

SCREENING/DIAGNOSIS

Understanding the relationship between chronic pain and cognition is important in recognizing signs of abuse or dependence. Persons with pain and comorbid depression are at a significantly higher risk of narcotic abuse and adverse events.[5–7] A study using real-time functional MRI showed that afferent pain pathways are altered by emotions and the state of the individual's attention.[5] Comorbid negative emotions (eg,

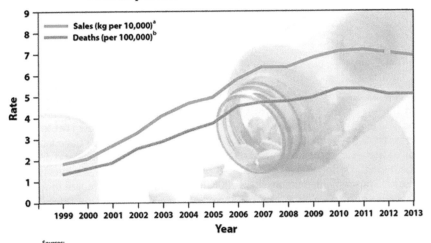

Sources:
[a]Automation of Reports and Consolidated Orders System (ARCOS) of the Drug Enforcement Administration (DEA), 2012 data not available.
[b]Centers for Disease Control and Prevention. National Vital Statistics System mortality data. (2015) Available from URL:
http://www.cdc.gov/nchs/deaths.htm.

Fig. 1. Trend of painkiller prescriptions related to deaths associated with use. (*From* Centers for Disease Control and Prevention. National Vital Statistics System. Mortality data. Available at: http://www.cdc.gov/nchs/deaths.htm. Accessed July 6, 2015.)

anger, sadness) heightened the afferent, reactionary pain pathways and interrupted the descending modulatory systems associated with pain relief and coping.[5,7,8] Emotional state and perception of pain were also shown to activate the same brain areas, such as the primary and secondary somatosensory cortex (S1, S2), anterior cingulate cortex, insula, prefrontal cortex, thalamus, and cerebellum.[5]

This relationship between emotional state and chronic pain has created difficulties for physicians caring for individuals who have both. Patients with chronic pain and co-morbid mental illness present challenges. As noted before, mental illness can increase intensity of pain and extend its duration by interrupting pain-modulating systems, but it can also increase risk for disability, drug abuse, and pain-seeking behavior, all leading to poorer outcomes (**Box 1**).[5,7]

Knowing this connection, physicians can screen for depression, substance abuse, and other mental illnesses using evidence-based tools intended to be a time-efficient method for identifying potential risk.[1,4] Common tools for screening used in the primary care setting include the Patient Health Questionnaire (PHQ) (**Fig. 2**) for depression and the Alcohol Use Disorders Identification Test-C (AUDIT-C) (**Box 2**) to identify substance abuse. The PHQ is a survey filled out by the patient, rating the frequency with which a patient experiences common signs of depression. This tool is rated based on gender, and scored to determine a positive result.[3,4]

The AUDIT-C is a screening tool to help identify alcohol abuse. This quick, 3-question survey gathers information about how much and how often an individual drinks alcohol.[1,3,4] Using the AUDIT-C along with asking the patient about use of illicit drugs can help physicians recognize a potential risk of narcotic dependence or pain-seeking behavior, and also help develop a treatment plan most appropriate for the patient.[4]

Taking an in-depth past medical history and performing a detailed physical examination can also provide insight into the potential risk of abuse and adverse events.[1,3,4] Patients with a history of any form of abuse, mental illness, or substance abuse may be at increased risk. In addition, those patients showing an exaggerated response to stimuli during physical examination should be of concern. The Centers for Disease Control and Prevention (CDC) have listed several potential red flags in treating pain with narcotic medications, including[3]:

- History of mental illness
- History of abuse (physical, emotional, or sexual)
- History of substance abuse
- Exaggerated somatic response noted during physical examination

---

Box 1
Effects of comorbid mental illness on chronic pain

- Increased pain intensity
- Decreased activity of descending pain-modulating systems
- Increased disability and poor outcomes
- Increased risk for substance abuse and adverse events
- Increased health care use

Data from Glombiewski J, Hartwich-Tersek J, Rief W. Depression in chronic back pain patients: prediction of pain intensity and pain disability in cognitive-behavioral treatment. Psychosomatics 2010;51(2):130–6.

Patient's name: _____   Date: _____

Over the past two weeks, how often have you been bothered by any of the following problems? (For each question, circle the number that represents the best answer.)

	Not at all	Several days	More than one half of the days	Nearly every day
1. Little interest or pleasure in doing things	0	1	2	3
2. Feeling down, depressed, or hopeless	0	1	2	3
3. Trouble falling asleep or staying asleep, or sleeping too much	0	1	2	3
4. Feeling tired or having little energy	0	1	2	3
5. Poor appetite or overeating	0	1	2	3
6. Feeling bad about yourself—or that you are a failure or have let yourself or your family down	0	1	2	3
7. Trouble concentrating on things such as reading the newspaper or watching television	0	1	2	3
8. Moving or speaking so slowly that other people have noticed. Or the opposite—being so fidgety or restless that you have been moving around a lot more than usual	0	1	2	3
9. Thoughts that you would be better off dead or of hurting yourself in some way	0	1	2	3

If you have had any of these problems, how difficult have they made it for you to do your work, take care of things at home, or get along with other people?

Not difficult at all	Somewhat difficult	Very difficult	Extremely difficult

Scoring instructions: The total PHQ-9 score is the sum of the scores for the responses to questions 1 through 9.

Interpreting the score to determine severity of depression:
0 to 4 = no symptoms or minimal symptoms
5 to 9 = minor symptoms
10 to 14 = moderate symptoms
15 to 19 = moderate to severe symptoms
20 or more = severe symptoms

Previously used criteria for diagnosing depression:
1. Depression diagnosis = symptoms frequency of "more than one half of the days" or "nearly every day" for Question 1 or 2 and
   Five or more of questions 3 through 9 (question 9 counts if answer is "several days" or more often).
   These criteria have a sensitivity of 73 percent and a specificity of 96 percent for depression.
2. PHQ-9 score ≥ 10. This score has a sensitivity of 88 percent and a specificity of 88 percent for depression.

Fig. 2. PHQ-9. (*Developed by* Drs. Robert L. Spitzer, Janet B.W. Williams, Kurt Kroenke and colleagues, with an educational grant from Pfizer Inc. No permission required to reproduce, translate, display or distribute.)

Screening patients for mental illness and substance abuse before initiating treatment with high-risk medications, as well as frequent rescreening during ongoing therapy, can help decrease the risk of adverse events and poor outcomes.[1,3,4]

MANAGEMENT GOALS

An important rule of thumb for clinicians to remember when treating patients with chronic pain is that the goal of care is not to eliminate an individual's pain. The goal of management is to promote the acceptance of chronic pain, to provide support and help maintain a healthy mood, and to promote independence in completing activities of daily living and sustaining gainful employment.[1,7,9]

Box 2
AUDIT-C example

AUDIT-C questionnaire for detecting alcoholism

1. How often do you have a drink containing alcohol?
   a. Never
   b. Monthly or less
   c. 2 to 4 times a month
   d. 2 to 3 times a week
   e. 4 or more times a week

2. How many standard drinks containing alcohol do you have on a typical day?
   a. 1 or 2
   b. 3 or 4
   c. 5 or 6
   d. 7 to 9
   e. 10 or more

3. How often do you have 6 or more drinks on 1 occasion?
   a. Never
   b. Less than monthly
   c. Monthly
   d. Weekly
   e. Daily or almost daily

The AUDIT-C is scored on a scale of 0 to 12.
Each AUDIT-C question has 5 answer choices. Points allotted are: a, 0 points; b, 1 points; c, 2 points; d, 3 points; e, 4 points.
Men: a score of 4 or more is considered positive; optimal for identifying hazardous drinking or active alcohol use disorders.
Women: a score of 3 or more is considered positive; optimal for identifying hazardous drinking or active alcohol use disorders.
   AUDIT-C is available for use in the public domain.

Some patients continue to experience pain long term, with difficulties returning to their baseline level of function. This clinical picture is identified as chronic pain syndrome, and is defined as pain not responding well to treatment and lasting longer than reasonably expected.[1,7,9–11] These patients pose a particular difficulty for primary care physicians managing this syndrome, because they often fail traditional therapies and become dependent on higher doses of medication treatments.[1,5,7,9,10,12]

PHARMACOLOGIC STRATEGIES

The potential risk for patients taking prescription narcotic medications has become widely publicized, but clinicians must remember that no analgesic is without risk and all should be used with caution. First-line treatment of pain usually begins with a nonsteroidal antiinflammatory, acetaminophen, an antiepileptic, or any combination of these medications. Guidelines for each medication's use, as well as specific contraindications, must be considered as part of the clinician's decision making.[1]

Prescription narcotic pain medications are appropriate when other pharmacologic and nonpharmacologic strategies have failed, or when there are contraindications to their use. Narcotics have an important role in the treatment of pain and, when used appropriately, they can serve to significantly improve quality of life. Any time a high-risk medication is prescribed, care must be taken to help maintain patient safety and prevent adverse events, such as an overdose or lethal drug combination. Several principles for narcotic prescribing can help allow for early intervention in cases of dependence or abuse, as well as discontinuation of unnecessary narcotic medications, and should be followed:

- Using the lowest effective dose in controlling pain
- Using long-acting formulas when the treatment will be prolonged
- Attempting frequent wean trials when appropriate
- Monitoring often for signs of dependence or abuse[1,3]

Also, if available, pain management specialists can be consulted to assist in treating pain that is refractory to conventional methods of treatment.[1]

NONPHARMACOLOGIC STRATEGIES

Given the intimate connection between chronic pain and cognition, cognitive behavior therapy and mindfulness techniques have been shown to help control and restructure the maladaptive cognitions and behaviors seen with chronic pain syndrome. The ultimate goal of this therapy is to help individuals living with chronic pain develop a more effective reaction to their pain through the use of techniques meant to inspire 4 realizations and dispel maladaptive cognitions/behaviors[7,9,13]:

1. Individuals are active interpreters of information, and make sense of stimuli through thought patterns developed through reactions from previous stimuli and subsequent consequence, whether positive or negative.
2. Individuals are responsible for their own thoughts and perceptions (ie, beliefs, thought patterns, negative or positive regard) and the subsequent behavior.
3. Thoughts and perceptions can modulate individuals' physiologic arousal and sensitivity to pain.
4. Tools for self-management are essential to well-being and resiliency.

Restructuring maladaptive behaviors requires setting realistic goals of treatment and dispelling misinformation.[7,12,14]

Two common maladaptive behaviors noted in chronic pain syndrome are catastrophic thinking and fear avoidance or guarding. Catastrophic thinking (**Table 2**)

Table 2	
Explanation of catastrophic thinking patterns	
Catastrophic Thinking Styles	**Explanation**
All or nothing	If something is not perfect, it is a failure
Disqualifying the positive	Disqualifying accomplishments and focusing on perceived failures
Jumping to conclusions	Mind reading and fortune telling
Emotional reasoning	Assuming emotions define an individual
Magnification	Exaggerating things out of proportion
Minimization	Making something seem less important than it should be
Labeling	Assigning labels to others or within
Criticizing	Using words like "must" or "should" inspires guilt and a sense of failure
Personalization	Displacing blame within or onto another person

Data from Borkum J. Maladaptive cognitions and chronic pain: epidemiology, neurobiology, and treatment. J Rat-Emo Cognitive Behav Ther 2010;28:4–24; and Farrugia D, Fetter H. Chronic pain: biological understanding and treatment suggestions for mental health counselors. J Ment Health Couns 2009;31(3):189–200.

consists of several dysfunctional thought patterns and contents. These thought patterns are common in individuals at high risk for poor outcomes. These thought patterns are destructive to individuals' sense of self-worth and can distort people's perception of ideal self and expectations. Approaching this restructuring of thought patterns as a change in behavior, using techniques such as motivational interviewing, can help patients dispel misinformation and encourage positive self-regard.[6,9]

Fear-avoidance behavior is another destructive coping mechanism that can lead to withdrawing from friends, family, and activities secondary to fear of pain or embarrassment. This behavior can trigger increased disability through a self-perpetuating cycle of trying to accomplish more than is reasonably expected and then needing prolonged periods of time to recuperate. These periods of inactivity often lead to stiffness and increased pain with resumption of activity (**Fig. 3**).[6,9]

Cognitive behavior therapy can be structured for use in the primary care setting, and has been shown to be effective in management of chronic pain.[12–19] When initiating therapy and for more difficult patients, frequent follow-up visits are important in establishing the groundwork for a more effective response to chronic pain. Combating catastrophic thinking can be achieved through journaling and recording events during which dysfunctional thought processes were experienced. This technique creates scope for dialogue between provider and patient on specific fears, with opportunity to reflect on the likelihood of serious catastrophe and to restructure destructive thought patterns while encouraging realization of resourcefulness and resiliency.[6,9,13]

SELF-MANAGEMENT STRATEGIES

Maintaining a healthy diet and prioritizing regular exercise is the recipe for well-being for any individual, but it is especially important for those managing life with chronic pain. Focused stretching modalities, such as therapeutic yoga and strength-building exercise help to maintain function and baseline activity level. There are free videos and a variety of resources that can be accessed online.[1]

The ultimate role of cognitive behavior therapy in chronic pain is to teach self-management tools that significantly improve quality of life by keeping patients active longer and restoring a sense of fulfillment.[6,16] An important and effective coping

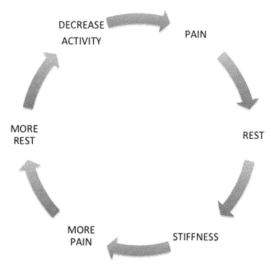

Fig. 3. The destructive cycle of chronic pain. (*Data from* Refs.[6,9,13])

Pain Diary

For each time slot write down what you were doing and how much pain you were in

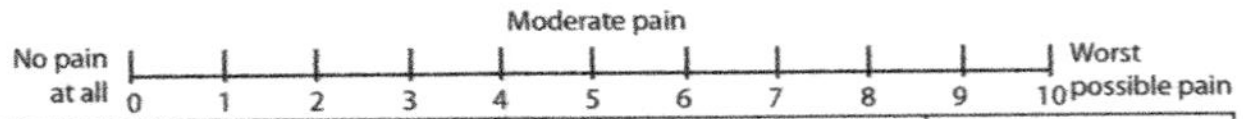

No pain at all |0 1 2 3 4 5 6 7 8 9 10| Worst possible pain

Moderate pain

	Monday	Tuesday	Wednesday	Thursday	Friday	Saturday	Sunday
7 AM to 9 AM							
9 AM to 10 AM							
10 AM to 11 AM							
11 AM to 12 PM							
12 to 1							
1 to 2							
2 to 3							
3 to 4							
4 to 5							
5 to 6							
6 to 7							
7 to 8							
8 to 9							
9 to 10							
10 to 12 AM							

Fig. 4. Pain diary. (*From* Psychology Tools. Available at: http://psychology.tools/. Accessed July 6, 2015; with permission.)

mechanism in chronic pain is pacing. Pacing recognizes that more can be accomplished in the long run if tasks are divided into reasonably timed phases to avoid the necessity of a prolonged resting period. An objective method to keep track of progress is a pain diary and a task planning/achievement chart (**Fig. 4**). A pain diary tracks the patient's level of pain throughout the day, giving the patient an opportunity to reflect on the level of pain during different times of day and in different scenarios. This diary can also be used for task planning, in order to set aside appropriate times during the day for activity and subsequent rest. The goal is to avoid fatigue and deterioration of pain.[1,6,16]

Another effective coping mechanism in the management of chronic pain is relaxation. Stress can lead to increased inflammation, increased muscle tension and spasm, as well as hypersensitivity to pain. Mindfulness techniques such as focused breathing and progressive muscle relaxation can help relieve stress and prevent worsening of pain and disability.[6,17,20]

Focused breathing (**Fig. 5**) involves patients keeping their attention focused on the timing and movement of respiration. This mindfulness technique modulates activity in the sympathetic nervous system, decreases levels of stress hormones, and has been shown to be beneficial in a myriad of chronic illnesses such as mood disorders (depression, anxiety, posttraumatic stress disorder), substance abuse, hypertension, lung disease, and chronic pain. Focused breathing can be used in conjunction with progressive muscle relaxation (**Fig. 6**) as an effective self-management tool in living with chronic pain. This technique of following a sequence of controlled muscle activation and relaxation has been shown to be especially beneficial in scenarios in which muscle spasm and spasticity predominate, such as migraine, multiple sclerosis, and neck/back pain, as well as neuropathy and restless leg syndrome. Patients should be counseled to discontinue using these techniques and schedule a follow-up visit if any of these techniques cause an increase in pain.[4,5,17,21]

Adequate sleep is essential in the management of chronic pain. Poor sleep decreases resiliency to pain and makes it more difficult to manage day-to-day business. Patients become less active, which often leads to a decreased functional baseline and increased

Mindfulness Techniques: Abdominal Breathing

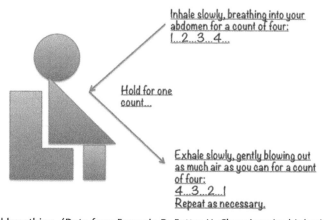

Inhale slowly, breathing into your abdomen for a count of four:
1...2...3...4...

Hold for one count...

Exhale slowly, gently blowing out as much air as you can for a count of four:
4...3...2...1
Repeat as necessary.

Fig. 5. Focused breathing. (*Data from* Farrugia D, Fetter H. Chronic pain: biological understanding and treatment suggestions for mental health counselors. J Ment Health Couns 2009;31(3):189–200; and Psychology Tools. Available at: http://psychology.tools. Accessed July 6, 2015.)

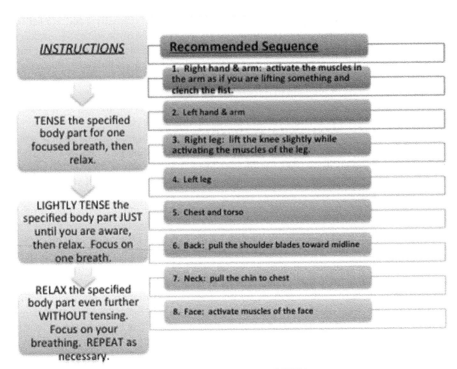

Fig. 6. Progressive muscle relaxation. (*Data from* Refs.[5,6,22,24])

risk for depression and substance abuse. Establishing good sleep hygiene helps manage fatigue and baseline activity level, and helps maintain quality of life (**Table 3**).[13,20,22]

Using these techniques regularly can help increase activity and build stamina, leading to decreased disability, increased self-worth, and significantly improved quality of life (**Fig. 7**).[20,22]

EVALUATION, ADJUSTMENT, RECURRENCE

Regular follow-up and consistent monitoring of progress are essential for effectively managing chronic pain. Scheduling 4-week to 6 week follow-up appointments is

Table 3
Guidelines for good sleep hygiene

Guidelines for Better Sleep	
Good for Sleep	Bad for Sleep
• Exercise regularly	• Napping
• Journaling	• Watching television in bed
• Focused breathing and progressive muscle relaxation	• Using a device with a bright screen within an hour before bed
• Establishing a bedtime routine	• Consuming caffeine in excess or after 6 PM
• Establishing an environment for sleep	• Consuming alcohol
	• Staying in bed when you cannot go to sleep

Data from Refs.[5,6,22,24]

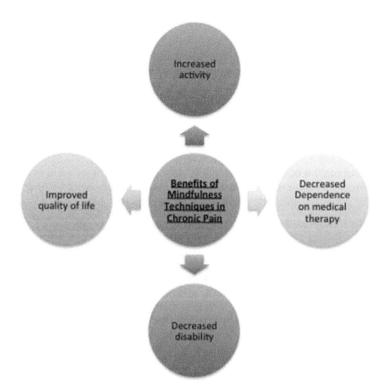

Fig. 7. Benefits of mindfulness therapy for chronic pain. (*Data from* Carlson L. Mindfulness-based interventions for physical conditions: a narrative review evaluating levels of evidence. ISRN Psychiatry 2012;2012:651583; and Kowal J, Wilson KG, Geck CM, et al. Changes in perceived pain severity during interdisciplinary treatment for chronic pain. Pain Res Manag 2011;16(6):451–6.)

common while establishing the groundwork for changing catastrophic thought patterns and teaching mindfulness techniques. Self-management techniques must be reinforced and encouraged frequently during the first stage of treatment, and patients must believe that they have an open dialogue on progress, barriers, and setbacks. Timing of maintenance visits is individualized and depends on adjunct medical therapy, comorbidities, and severity of disease. Regular screening for depression and substance use is recommended at each maintenance visit to allow for early intervention with mental health issues. Physical therapy and focused stretching modalities, such as therapeutic yoga, should be considered important parts of treatment in exacerbations of chronic pain–causing conditions and used whenever appropriate. For patients who require medical therapy with opioids, maintenance visits are recommended at least every 3 months. Dosage monitoring to achieve the lowest effective dosage, as well as screening for misuse and abuse, is strongly encouraged at each visit. Discontinuing opioids quickly after surgery or acute injury is essential for preventing dependence.[1,3,23]

Physicians who prescribe opioids must take care to protect patients from misuse and adverse events. A written contract between the prescribing physician and the patient, called a controlled medication agreement, is necessary for regulating use. These contracts establish guidelines for medical therapy and agreed-on goals of care, including consistent pharmacy for easy refill monitoring, avoidance of illicit drugs, informed consent on random drug testing, consistent refill timing, required maintenance visits, and appropriate treatment of staff. Also, most states have prescription-monitoring programs that routinely track prescriptions for Schedule II medications. Registering for these programs is required for prescribing controlled medications in most states, and use can alert physicians to dependence or fraudulent activity by identifying patients who are getting medications with a high abuse potential from multiple providers. Most abused prescriptions originate with what was thought to be a legitimate prescription, and liability is high for physicians who encounter an adverse event.[1,23]

Physical therapy and focused stretching modalities, such as therapeutic yoga, should be considered important parts of treatment in exacerbations of chronic pain–causing conditions. During exacerbations, assessing triggering events or injuries can give insight into a potential plan for prevention of future flares. Also, screening for new-onset mental health issues and reiteration of self-management techniques, such as pacing, help patients maintain baseline well-being and prepare for future exacerbations.[4,12,14]

SUMMARY/DISCUSSION

Management of pain is common in primary care. In some of these patients, pain is an ever-present component of their chronic illness. Physicians are realizing that opioid medications are overused in the treatment of non–cancer-related pain, and that the consequences have been severe, with deaths related to opioid medications increasing, forcing physicians to look for safer alternatives for treatment. With the understanding that individuals' emotional states can change how they perceive pain, cognitive behavior therapy and mindfulness techniques should play an important role in the management of pain. Healthy diet, physical therapy, stress reduction, and combating catastrophic thought patterns through behavioral therapy can help patients avoid chronic pain and disability through maintaining a higher level of functioning and resiliency toward pain.

Cognitive behavior therapy works to restructure maladaptive thought processes, such as overgeneralization or labeling, and helps to build more effective coping mechanisms. This therapy can help patients accept their chronic pain, set realistic goals for management, and continue to maintain quality of life. Reflecting tools, such as journaling, and maintaining an open dialogue can help patients gain insight into triggers and adapt to new limitations. Self-management assessment tools and mindfulness techniques aid patients with monitoring their own progress, pacing to stay active, and achieving stress reduction. Good sleep hygiene should also be encouraged to maintain resiliency and level of function.

If prescription opioid medications are required for treatment, care must be taken to ensure patient safety and to decrease liability for prescribers. Using the lowest effective dose of opioid, instituting initial and follow-up screening for depression or substance use, and adjusting to safer formulations when long-term opioids are necessary can help avoid poor outcomes. Establishing a medication agreement with patients on opioids, and taking steps to maintain a safe prescribing practice, can also help avoid liability for prescribers. State-issued prescription-monitoring programs aid physicians in identifying patients involved in fraudulent behavior such as receiving prescriptions for controlled substances from multiple prescribers. Substance abuse treatment programs and strategies should be used in these scenarios of misuse or abuse.

Recommendations for the management of pain in primary care are trending away from the use of highly addictive and often abused medications and toward using the cognitive connection to pain to help patients accept and self-manage their conditions.

REFERENCES

1. American Academy of Pain Medicine. AAPM facts and figures on pain. 2011. Available at: http://www.painmed.org/patientcenter/facts_on_pain.aspx#refer. Accessed July 6, 2015.
2. Arnold I, de Waal MW, Eekhof JA, et al. Medically unexplained physical symptoms in primary care: A controlled study on the effectiveness of cognitive-behavioral treatment by the family physician. Psychosomatics 2009;50(5):515–24.
3. Centers for Disease Control (CDC). Available at: www.cdc.gov. Accessed July 6, 2015.
4. McCracken L, Thompson M. Components of mindfulness in patients with chronic pain. J Psychopathol Behav Assess 2008;31:75–82.
5. Bushnell M, Ceko M, Law L. Cognitive and emotional control of pain and its disruption in chronic pain. Nat Rev Neurosci 2013;14:502–11.
6. Farrugia D, Fetter H. Chronic pain: Biological understanding and treatment suggestions for mental health counselors. J Ment Health Counsel 2009;31(3): 189–200.
7. Glombiewski J, Hartwich-Tersek J, Rief W. Depression in chronic back pain patients: Prediction of pain intensity and pain disability in cognitive-behavioral treatment. Psychosomatics 2010;51(2):130–6.
8. Trafton J, Sorrell JT, Holodniy M, et al. Outcomes associated with a cognitive-behavioral chronic pain management program implemented in three public HIV primary care clinics. J Behav Health Serv Res 2012;39(2):158–73.
9. Borkum J. Maladaptive cognitions and chronic pain: epidemiology, neurobiology, and treatment. J Rat-Emo Cognitive Behav Ther 2010;28:4–24.
10. Committee on Advancing Pain Research, Care, and Education Board of Health Sciences Policy. Pain in America: Blueprint for transforming prevention, care, education, and research. Washington, DC: Institute of Medicine of the National Academies; 2011. Available at: http://iom.nationalacademies.org/Reports/2011/Relieving-Pain-in-America-A-Blueprint-for-Transforming-Prevention-Care-Education-Research.aspx.
11. Cully J, Armento ME, Mott J, et al. Brief cognitive behavioral therapy in primary care: a hybrid type 2 patient-randomized effectiveness-implementation program. Implementat Sci 2012;7(64):1–12.
12. Skinner M, Wilson H, Turk D. Cognitive-behavioral perspective and cognitive-behavioral therapy for people with chronic pain: distinction, outcomes, and innovations. J Cognit Psychother 2012;26(2):93–113.
13. Dennison L, Moss-Morris R. Cognitive-behavioral therapy: what benefits can it offer people with multiple sclerosis? Expert Rev Neurotherapy 2010;10(9): 1383–7.
14. Vazquez-Rivera S, González-Blanch C, Rodríguez-Moya L, et al. Brief cognitive-behavioral therapy with fibromyalgia patients in routine care. Compr Psychiatry 2009;50:517–25.
15. Garmon B, Philbrick J, Becker D, et al. Mindfulness-based stress reduction for chronic pain: A systematic review. J Pain Management 2014;7(1):23–36.
16. Hofmann S, Asnaani A, Vonk IJ, et al. The efficacy of cognitive behavioral therapy: a review of meta-analyses. Cognit Ther Res 2012;36:427–40.
17. Ussher M, Spatz A, Copland C, et al. Immediate effects of a brief mindfulness-based body scan on patients with chronic pain. J Behav Med 2014;37:127–34.
18. Woltmann E, Grogan-Kaylor A, Perron B, et al. Comparative effectiveness of collaborative chronic care models for mental health conditions across primary,

specialty, and behavioral health care settings: systematic review and meta-analysis. Am J Psychiatry 2012;169:790–804.

19. White J. CBT and the challenge of primary care: developing effective, efficient, equitable, acceptable and accessible services for common mental health problems. J Public Ment Health 2009;7(1):32–41.

20. Kowal J, Wilson KG, Geck CM, et al. Changes in perceived pain severity during interdisciplinary treatment for chronic pain. Pain Res Manag 2011;16(6):451–6.

21. Sipe W, Eisendrath S. Mindfulness-based cognitive theory: theory and practice. Can J Psychiatry 2012;57(2):63–9.

22. Carlson L. Mindfulness-based interventions for physical conditions: a narrative review evaluating levels of evidence. ISRN Psychiatry 2012;2012:651583.

23. Substance Abuse and Mental Health Services Administration (SAMHSA). Available at: www.samhsa.gov. Accessed July 6, 2015.

24. Psychology Tools. Available at: http://psychology.tools. Accessed July 6, 2015.

Substance Abuse Screening and Treatment

Johnny C. Tenegra, MD, MS*, Bobby Leebold, LCSW

KEYWORDS

- Substance abuse disorder • Substance misuse • Screening • Substitution therapies
- Blocking therapies

KEY POINTS

- Although the prevalence of substance use disorders in primary care patients runs high, physicians, due to lack of adequate training and skepticism about treatment effectiveness, feel unprepared to tackle substance abuse disorders in the office.
- Diagnosis of a substance abuse disorder can be made through a combination of history taking, screening questionnaires, physical examination, and chemical testing.
- Primary care physicians are well-positioned to treat those with substance abuse with knowledge and access to behavioral techniques, community resources, and pharmacologic strategies.
- The correlation of substance use disorders with other medical and psychiatric comorbidities makes the treatment of substance use disorders all the more important to patient care.

INTRODUCTION

The role of a primary care physician in the management of substance use disorders can be complex and challenging. The scope of the problem is significant and underscores a public health epidemic. In 2013, an estimated 24.6 million Americans aged 12 or older were current illicit drug users, representing 9.4% of the population.[1] In the general population, roughly 15.5 million were dependent on or abused alcohol alone, with some 100,000 people dying each year in the United States as a result.[2] Furthermore, in 2004, it was estimated that more than 9.4% of Americans older than the age of 12 had a full-blown drug or alcohol addiction.[3]

The issue is made even more complicated by the increase in the nonmedicinal use of both prescription and over-the-counter (OTC) medications. This problem is particularly prevalent among adolescents, in whom the use of these drugs has steadily escalated over the past few years. The most common drugs of choice include stimulants, sedatives, tranquilizers, and most notably, specific analgesics such as opioids.

Decatur Family Medicine Residency, Southern Illinois University School of Medicine, 102 West Kenwood Avenue, Suite 100, Decatur, IL 62526, USA
* Corresponding author.
E-mail address: jtenegra@siumed.edu

Prim Care Clin Office Pract 43 (2016) 217–227
http://dx.doi.org/10.1016/j.pop.2016.01.008
0095-4543/16/$ – see front matter © 2016 Elsevier Inc. All rights reserved.
primarycare.theclinics.com

The abuse of OTC medications is equally problematic with teens and young adults abusing cough and cold medications. In a 2006 survey, 3.1 million persons aged 12 to 25 used an OTC cough and cold medication to get high.[4]

Research estimates that between 20% and 26% of primary care patients suffer from a substance use disorder.[5] The indicated prevalence must be considered in light of the fact that most of those with a substance use disorder do not seek out treatment in the substance abuse treatment system. The result is that the primary care physician becomes the first potential provider to recognize the problem and begin to address the issue with the patient. The importance of doing so cannot be trivialized because these disorders consistently rank among the 10 leading preventable risk factors for years of life lost to death and disability.[6] In addition, substance abuse disorders are associated with a higher risk of a variety of conditions, including hypertension, congestive heart failure, cirrhosis of the liver, lower back pain, arthritis, hepatitis C, pneumonia, chronic obstructive pulmonary disease, along with injuries and overdoses associated with misuse. Furthermore, substance use disorders are also responsible for the complication of many other medical conditions, contributing to the increasing cost associated with the health care system. Americans pay nearly $1000 annually to cover the costs of unnecessary health care, extra law enforcement, motor vehicle crashes, crime, and lost productivity due to substance abuse.[7]

Despite the impact illicit substances has on health care, physicians report low levels of preparedness to recognize and help patients with substance use disorders. Physicians cite a lack of adequate training in medical school, residency, and continuing education courses. Physicians also report skepticism about treatment effectiveness, time constraints, perceived patient resistance, discomfort with discussing substance abuse, and fear of losing patients. Patient self-report supports this information. In one study, 43% of patients said their physician never diagnosed their addiction, and 11% reported that the physician knew about their addiction, but did nothing about it.[8]

With this information in mind, the goal of this article is to briefly discuss the screening, diagnosis, management, and treatment of substance abuse, one of the more complicated and challenging public health issues faced by primary care physicians.

SCREENING/DIAGNOSIS

Despite modern medicine's many advances, detecting substance abuse problems has continued to challenge primary care providers. Screening is a vital first step, and many organizations, including the American Medical Association, recommend that clinicians routinely ask patients about substance use. Screening for a substance abuse problem relies heavily on asking the right questions. When the correct questions are asked, research has shown that the odds of successfully uncovering substance abuse in a general clinical setting can be improved significantly. There are numerous screening tools at the disposal of the primary care physician. In later discussion is a select sampling of the more popular measures used in the primary care setting.

Developed by the World Health Organization, the Alcohol Use Disorders Identification Test assesses alcohol consumption, drinking behaviors, and alcohol-related problems. This short, 10-item questionnaire is particularly suitable for use in primary care settings, has both a clinician-administered and a self-report version, and can been used with a variety of populations and cultural groups. The clinician-administered version should be administered by a health professional or paraprofessional.[9]

Modeled after the widely used Michigan Alcoholism Screening Test,[10] The Drug Abuse Screening Test (DAST) includes a 10-item (DAST-10) and a 20-item (DAST-20) brief screening tool to assess specifically for nonalcohol drug use. One of the fastest drug abuse screening tools around, each question requires a yes or no response and can be administered by a clinician or self-administered to both adults and older youth. This tool can be particularly useful in its ability to address the increasing epidemic of prescription drug abuse.

The CAGE-AID (Cut down, Annoyed, Guilty, Eye-opener, Adapted to Include Drugs) questionnaire is a 4-item tool that takes 4 minutes or less to administer and is used to assess for drug/alcohol use problems in adults and adolescents (older than 16 years). The CAGE-AID questions focus on the behavioral effects of alcohol or drug use with higher scores indicating the need for the physician to ask more specific questions about frequency and quantity. This tool is good for health care professionals because it is easy to remember and can be administered by an interviewer, self-administered in pencil-and-paper format, or computer administered.

Knowing the type of agent involved in a substance use disorder is important for creating a management plan for the patient. Classes of substances used include stimulants, hallucinogens, and depressants. At times, the patient may only know a substance by street name. Many of the substances that are abused have their own profiles of symptoms but may share similar signs and symptoms with other drugs within the same class (**Table 1**).

To confirm the patient's drug of use, laboratory testing is a useful tool in screening patients for substance use disorders. However, in itself, it is not diagnostic. A multitude of modalities are used to screen patients for substance abuse, with the versatility of each modality increasing. Each one has their own advantages and disadvantages, including how easy it is to adulterate (**Table 2**). Urine testing is most widely used because of its availability, cost, and rapid results. It is helpful to keep in mind that common medications ingested by patients may cause false positives, and a correlation between the patient's history and physical diagnosis will help with diagnosing these.

Table 1
Profiles of signs and symptoms of intoxication and withdrawal of selected drugs

Substance	Intoxication	Withdrawal
Cocaine	Pupillary dilation, hypertension, cocaine bug hallucinations	"Crash" includes depression, fatigue, malaise, craving
Amphetamines	Pupillary dilation, hypertension, prolonged wakefulness	"Crash" includes depression, lethargy, stomach cramps, hunger
Alcohol	Loss of inhibition, labile moods, blackouts	Tachycardia, hypertension, delirium tremens
Opioids	Pinpoint pupils, nausea, vomiting, seizures	Anxiety, sweating, fever, diarrhea, yawning
Barbiturates/ benzodiazepines	Respiratory depression	Anxiety, seizures, tremors, insomnia
Phencyclidine (PCP)	Belligerence, fever, nystagmus, ataxia, fever	Depression, restlessness, thoughts and sleep disturbances
Marijuana	Euphoria, delusions, slowed time, increased appetite	Irritability, depression, nausea

Data from Kowalchuk A, Reed B. Substance use disorders. In: Rakel RE, Rakel D, editors. Textbook of family medicine. 9th edition. New York: Elsevier Saunders; 2016. p. 1159.e1; and Detoxification and Substance Abuse Treatment. No. 45. Center for Substance Abuse Treatment. Rockville (MD): Substance Abuse and Mental Health Services Administration (US); 2006.

Table 2
Strengths and weaknesses of different laboratory testing for substance abuse

Test	Tests Available	Advantages	Disadvantages
Breath	Alcohol	Immediate results	Blood levels needed for medical management, if needed
Blood	Most drugs	Difficult to manipulate, accurate, can detect recent ingestion	Drugs can clear quickly compared with urine; slightly invasive
Hair	Cocaine, marijuana, opiates, amphetamines, PCP	Noninvasive, detects patterns of use over time due to longest duration of positivity	Not widely available, drug or metabolite amounts may vary with hair color; difficult to process
Saliva	Amphetamines, alcohol, methamphetamines, opiates, cocaine, marijuana, PCP	Immediate results	Qualitative result only
Sweat (PharmChek sweat patch)	Cocaine, heroin, codeine, synthetic opiates, amphetamines, PCP, marijuana	Noninvasive, using patch	Quantification of drug levels difficult
Urine	Most drugs	Noninvasive, longer duration of positivity, rapid results, low cost	Easy to adulterate, collection is usually observed

Data from Kowalchuk A, Reed B. Substance use disorders. In: Rakel RE, Rakel D, editors. Textbook of family Medicine. 9th edition. New York: Elsevier Saunders; 2016. p. 1156; and Gwyther RE. Addiction. In: Essentials of family medicine. 3rd edition. New York; Baltimore (MD): Williams & Wilkins; 1993. p. 248.

The Diagnostic and Statistical Manual of Mental Disorders, 5th edition (DSM-V) criteria can be used to stratify severity of substance use disorders.[11] Characteristics of substance use, such as craving and desire for substances, impairment of daily activities, and frequency of use, are a part of the DSM-V criteria. Based on the severity, primary care providers can make appropriate decisions on how to manage community resources for the care of these patients. Important changes from the DSM-IV criteria include dropping use of the terms substance abuse and substance dependence, along with a removal of legal problems from qualifying criteria, replaced by the criteria of craving. DSM-IV and DSM-V criteria have been shown to have a good correlation for multiple substances.[12] However, it is yet to be seen whether the new DSM-V criteria will have an impact on management and outcomes.[13]

MANAGEMENT GOALS

Referral to a substance use clinic is recommended for those with substance use disorders.[14] However, primary care physicians are unique in their position to screen, treat, and refer patients misusing substances. Once detected, the management of these patients is paramount throughout the continuum of care and involves specific goals and the interventions by which to achieve these goals. Management goals should flow from the screening, which determined misuse, abuse, or dependence and contain specific elements. They include the following[5]:

- *Developing a treatment plan* that not only identifies the substance misuse but also targets associated problems such as physical conditions related to the misuse, and potential psychosocial aspects related to the problematic usage. Furthermore, the plan should contain specific goals and strategies to complete these objectives, along with the techniques and services to be provided by identified specialists.
- *Periodic reassessment to evaluate the patient's needs*, especially as it pertains to psychosocial or mental health issues. For example, suicidal ideation should be carefully monitored and dealt with promptly should the issue arise.
- *Ongoing monitoring of progress, as it relates not only to response to treatment but also to the patient's overall physical health.* This monitoring should be conducted through written notes that report detailed information regarding treatment effectiveness, ongoing laboratory tests, and so on. In addition, this should include follow-up to determine if work with the patient's therapist or counselor is helping as well as to gauge treatment compliance and participation.
- *Providing education* to help the patient understand their diagnosis, its cause, and prognosis as well as the risks involved with treatment. This education should include not only the patient but also others involved in his or her treatment, which may include family and/or spouse.

PHARMACOLOGIC STRATEGIES

Pharmacologic agents (**Table 3**) may play a major role in the treatment of substance abuse and depend on the setting and acuity in which an abused drug is encountered as well as the type of drug used. Immediate reversal of the drug may be needed in acute circumstances when respiratory or cardiac status may be threatened. Pharmacologic therapy used to intervene with long-term substance abuse takes many forms, including receptor agonists, receptor antagonists, or slow taper of an agent to wean without withdrawal symptoms. The goals of pharmacologic therapy are to reduce consumption and prevent relapse of the use of the drug. Many of these treatments are combined with nonpharmacologic interventions, which are discussed later.

Table 3 Examples of pharmacologic strategies	
Substitution therapies	Methadone Buprenorphine Nicotine patches/gum
Blocking therapies	Naloxone Naltrexone
Triggered effect therapy	Disulfiram
Tapering therapy	Use with benzodiazepines

Data from Refs.[14–17]

Substitution Therapies

Substitution therapies include methadone and nicotine patches. With these therapies, the addictive agent is substituted in a different form. Methadone has improved the lives of many patients, but due to limited centers for distribution with resulting long waiting lists for required daily visits, patients may drive many miles to obtain this drug therapy. Buprenorphine is a partial agonist that comes in sublingual form by itself or in combination with naloxone, an opioid antagonist (Suboxone). Naloxone is only placed in the combination to prevent abuse of the therapy. Buprenorphine therapy has been proven to be safe and effective,[15,16] but can only be prescribed in office after training and receipt of a waiver from the Center for Substance Abuse Treatment and Drug Enforcement Administration.[14]

Another example of substitution therapy involves smoking cessation, wherein nicotine substitution is available in both transdermal patches and chewing gum. The patients are instructed to quit smoking on the day they start the treatment, with goal being reduction in the amount of nicotine intake over time through tapering doses.

Blocking Therapies

Blocking therapies are used quite frequently in acute and chronic cases of opiate abuse. Here, the medications are competitive agonists for the binding sites of the abused substances. Naloxone is used to reverse opiate overdose, whereas naltrexone is used in long-term use. Naltrexone is very popular for use in professionals who require monitoring for a licensing board. A strong motivator for naltrexone therapy is that relapse while on therapy can lead to losing a license to practice, leading to high success rates.[17]

Triggered Effect Therapies

Triggered effect therapies include disulfiram, which has been used in the past for alcohol abuse. By creating an accumulation of acetaldehyde, negative effects, such as nausea, vomiting, and vertigo, can be associated negatively with alcohol intake. Although previous literature had described disulfiram treatment falling out of favor, it recently has been shown that disulfiram may reduce drinking days and be effective at reducing chances of drinking in the short term.[18] Management with disulfiram requires patient compliance for effectiveness.

Tapering Therapy

Tapering therapy can be used with drugs such as benzodiazepines, where tapering is recommended over a several month period. This intervention is most successful in those who are highly motivated and can be trusted to frequently report back. Patients will be at risk of withdrawal symptoms, such as increased anxiety, depression, seizures, and altered mental status.[14]

NONPHARMACOLOGIC AND SELF-MANAGEMENT STRATEGIES

There is no single approach to treating and/or managing persons with a substance abuse disorder. Treatment strategies should be used while taking into consideration the diagnosis (misuse, abuse, or dependency/withdrawal) as well as any comorbidity. Moreover, equal importance must be given to addressing related social determinants of health associated with the substance abuse to improve outcomes, such as homelessness or unemployment. Before delving too deeply into specific treatment approaches, a brief discussion of the theoretic perspective as it relates to treatment is warranted. Current approaches reflect an integration of multiple models to address the problem. The following brief review can help primary care physicians understand the philosophic underpinnings of different treatment modalities, which include the following[5]:

1. The medical model: focuses on the physiologic causes of addiction. The emphasis is on the physician to use pharmacology as the primary means to alleviate symptoms and change behavior (methadone, for example, to treat withdrawal).
2. The psychological model: using a mental health professional, the emphasis is on emotional factors or learned patterns of maladaptive behavior (psychotherapy, for example).
3. The sociocultural model: changing the social, physical, and cultural environment to promote self-help through fellowship, spirituality, and social networks (Alcoholics Anonymous, for example).

Many times, a patient's journey to recovery and abstinence begins in the primary care physician's office. The first experience in identifying and addressing a patient's substance misuse is critical, due to not only its impact on treatment success but also the cost-conscious utilization of services while placing the patient in the least restrictive environment. As such, one of the tools that primary care physicians have at their disposal, which has demonstrated beneficial outcomes in the literature, is a brief intervention, which provides screening (CAGE questionnaire, for example), an assessment of the client's readiness to change, targeted intervention, and appropriate referral. The application of such a brief intervention model begins with a determination of hazardous, harmful, or dependent usage. Based on the results of the interview and the tool, primary care physicians are able to provide results, education, and recommendations to the patient to begin the change process. Below are listed the basic necessary components of a brief intervention[5]:

1. Give feedback about screening results, impairment, and risks while clarifying the findings.
2. Inform the patient about safe consumption limits and offer advice about change.
3. Assess the patient's readiness to change (see stages of change models).
4. Negotiate goals and strategies for change.
5. Arrange for follow-up treatment.
6. Referral for specialized treatment (if necessary).

Examples of brief interventions include the FRAMES Intervention Technique[19] (**Box 1**) and The Five "A's"[20] (**Box 2**). Brief interventions are best used with mild to moderate substance abuse as well as when apparent negative consequences due to current consumption are present. In addition, if comorbid conditions will be

---

Box 1
FRAMES intervention

Feedback about personal risk

Responsibility of the patient for change

Advice to change

Menu of strategies

Expression of empathy

Self-efficacy

Adapted from Miller WR, Sanchez VC. Motivating young adults for treatment and lifestyle change. In: Howard G, editor. Issues in alcohol use and misuse in young adults. Notre Dame (IN): University of Notre Dame Press; 1993.

---

exacerbated by substance misuse, or if the patient resists further outside assessment of recommended treatment, brief intervention within the primary care setting may be beneficial.[21] Another benefit of brief intervention is the ability to use it as a complement to, or in association with, ongoing specialized treatment. As the patient is able to demonstrate responsiveness, or lack thereof, to agreed on interventions, the treatment environment can be changed to more restrictive settings or can move in a less restrictive direction as indicated even if a more intensive treatment setting was initially agreed on. These settings include (from most intensive to least) inpatient hospitalization, residential treatment, intensive outpatient treatment, and outpatient treatment.

Inpatient hospitalization is the most restrictive and costly of these settings. Generally providing 24-hour around-the-clock care, this setting specializes in the medical management of detoxification using a multidisciplinary approach and is reserved typically for acute situations. Hospitalization is a short-term intensive approach lasting days to months and is used solely for the purpose of stabilizing the patient in order to move on to less restrictive care. Patients who have experienced a severe overdose, severe withdrawal symptoms, medical issues complicating withdrawal, a significant psychiatric comorbidity, or who are experiencing acute substance abuse and have not responded to other least restrictive forms of treatment are appropriate for this level of care.

Box 2
Five "A's" intervention (tobacco cessation example)

Ask: Identify and document tobacco use status for every patient at every visit.

Advise: In a clear, strong, and personalized manner, urge every tobacco user to quit.

Assess: Is the tobacco user willing to make a quit attempt at this time?

Assist: For the patient willing to make a quit attempt, use counseling and pharmacotherapy to help him or her quit.

Arrange: Schedule follow-up contact, in person, or by telephone, preferably within the first week after the quit date.

From Five Major Steps to Intervention (The "5 A's"). Agency for Healthcare Research and Quality, Rockville, MD. 2012. Available at: http://www.ahrq.gov/professionals/clinicians-providers/guidelines-recommendations/tobacco/5steps.html. Accessed October 1, 2015; with permission.

Residential treatment is the next level of care for patients who lack social support, who struggle with significant substance abuse problems, and who have tried other less restrictive environments and not been able to remain abstinent, but do not meet the criteria for hospitalization. These programs provide 24-hour supervision and are a live-in facility where treatment takes place via various modalities, including 12-step meetings, groups, individual therapy, and social skills training, along with treatment of psychological comorbidities. This particular modality tends to have better outcomes for certain patient populations, such as adolescents, for example, due in part to the change in environment.[22,23]

Intensive outpatient treatment, also known as partial hospitalization, can be the first transition from either a residential or an inpatient stay. This approach requires that the patient attend treatment typically during waking hours for 3 to 8 hours daily for up to 5 to 7 days per week. A full array of services is offered and is most suitable for patients with jobs and an extensive social network. Such patients may then transition to regular outpatient treatment whereby the same approaches are used, but in a more limited timeframe typically consisting of 1 to 2 visits one time weekly for 1 hour. This timeframe allows the patient to continue to focus on and reinforce treatment gains that were made in a more restrictive setting. Patients appropriate for this setting include those with significant motivation, transportation, and stable living arrangements. Treatment approaches used include group therapy and marital therapy, for example.

Increasingly, substance abuse/dependence is considered within an ongoing chronic disease framework with relapse always a possibility. As such, self-management for addictions is a vital treatment approach, encouraging the patient to take responsibility for their recovery by using resources within his or her environment and community.[24] Self-management allows the patient the autonomy to make treatment choices that will work for him or her with the goal of reducing misuse or maintaining abstinence. However, careful consideration must be made in regard to the individual patient's characteristics or circumstances because this approach is not for every patient. Such factors as unemployment, poverty, and lack of social support may make this a less desirable approach for patients experiencing these challenges. Involving oneself in Alcoholics Anonymous and other 12-step self-help and support group techniques are examples of this approach.

COMORBIDITIES AND RECURRENCE

Primary care clinicians need to be aware of comorbidities that are associated with substance use. Sexually transmitted diseases, such as human immunodeficiency virus, chlamydia, and gonorrhea, occur with increased frequency in patients with substance use.[13] Furthermore, intravenous drug users have their own set of comorbidities, including skin abscesses, cellulitis, infectious endocarditis, hepatitis, and pneumonia. Other mental health issues also run comorbid with substance use and must be addressed. In 2013, about 17.5% of adults (7.7 million) with any serious mental illness fit the criteria of substance use disorder.[1] Patients have an increased risk of a major depressive episode when using illicit drugs. In addition, clinicians should educate patients who are or will be considering pregnancy, because of the impact on fetal development many of these substances have.

Compliance with treatment plans for substance use disorders was found to be similar to other chronic medical illnesses, including hypertension, diabetes, and asthma.[25] The relapse rate of substance use disorders was also found to be similar to that of chronic illness, making ongoing support and monitoring with a primary care clinician crucial to successful treatment outcomes.[26]

SUMMARY

For primary care clinicians, substance abuse is an important aspect that must be addressed in taking care of the whole patient. With its relationship to other health conditions, substance use recognition and treatment are crucial to improved overall health for patients. Screening as well as anticipatory guidance during preventive visits can inform patients regarding the dangers of substance misuse/abuse, and treatment plans can integrate strategies to address these issues early on. With the multitude of screening tools, knowledge of the substances abused, and treatment resources and strategies, primary care physicians are well equipped to help their patients.

REFERENCES

1. Substance Abuse and Mental Health Services Administration. Results from the 2013 National Survey on Drug Use and Health: mental health findings. HHS Publication No. (SMA) 14–4887. Rockville (MD): Substance Abuse and Mental Health Services Administration; 2014.
2. Fact Sheets—Alcohol Use and Your Health. 2014. Available at: http://www.cdc.gov/alcohol/fact-sheets/alcohol-use.htm. Accessed October 1, 2015.
3. Substance Abuse and Mental Health Services Administration. Office of Applied Studies: results from the 2004 National Survey on Drug Use and Health: National Findings (NSDUH Series H-28, DHHS Publication No. SMA 05–4062). Rockville (MD): Department of Health and Human Services; 2005.
4. Alcohol, Tobacco, and Other Drugs. Substance Abuse and Mental Health Services Administration Web site. 2015. Available at: http://www.samhsa.gov/atod/other-drugs. Accessed November 1, 2015.
5. Center for Substance Abuse Treatment. A guide to substance abuse services for primary care clinicians. Treatment Improvement Protocol (TIP) Series, No. 24. Rockville (MD): Substance Abuse and Mental Health Services Administration (US); 1997.
6. Murray CJ, Atkinson C, Bjalla K, et al. The State of US Health, 1990-2010 burden of diseases, injuries, and risk factors. JAMA 2013;310:591–606.
7. Hall BP, Hawkinberry D, Moyers-Scott P. Prescription drug abuse & addiction: past, present and future: the paradigm for an epidemic. W V Med J 2010;106: 26–32.
8. CASA. The National Center on Substance Abuse at Columbia University. Missed opportunity: national survey of primary care physicians and patients on substance abuse. New York: National Center on Substance Abuse at Columbia University; 2000.
9. Screening and brief intervention for alcohol problems in primary health care. World Health Organization Web site. Available at: http://www.who.int/substance_abuse/activities/sbi/en/. Accessed October 1, 2015.
10. Selzer ML. The Michigan Alcoholism Screening Test (MAST): the quest for a new diagnostic instrument. Am J Psychiatry 1971;127:1653–8.
11. American Psychiatric Association. Diagnostic and statistical manual of mental disorders. 5th edition. Washington, DC: APA; 2013. Text revision (DSM-V).
12. Compton WM, Dawson DA, Goldstein RB, et al. Crosswalk between DSM-IV dependence and DSM-5 substance use disorders for opioids, cannabis, cocaine, and alcohol. Drug Alcohol Depend 2013;132:387–90.
13. Kowalchuk A, Reed B. Substance use disorders. In: Rakel RE, Rakel D, editors. Textbook of family medicine. 9th edition. New York: Elsevier Saunders; 2016. p. 1152–63.

14. Shapiro B, Coffa D, McCance-Katz EF. A primary care approach to substance misuse. Am Fam Physician 2013;88:113–21.
15. Ling W, Wesson DR. Clinical efficacy of buprenorphine: comparisons to methadone and placebo. Drug Alcohol Depend 2003;70(2 suppl):S49–57.
16. Mattick RP, Kimber J, Breen C, et al. Buprenorphine maintenance versus placebo or methadone maintenance for opioid dependence. Cochrane Database Syst Rev 2008;(2):CD002207.
17. Reading EG. Nine years' experience with chemically dependent physicians: the New Jersey experiences. Md Med J 1992;41(4):325–9.
18. Jorgensen CH, Pedersen B, Tonnesen H. The efficacy of disulfiram for the treatment of alcohol use disorder. Alcohol Clin Exp Res 2011;35:1749–58.
19. Miller WR, Sanchez VC. Motivating young adults for treatment and lifestyle change. In: Howard G, editor. Issues in alcohol use and misuse in young adults. Notre Dame (IN): University of Notre Dame Press; 1993. p. 55–81.
20. Five Major Steps to Intervention (The "5 A's"). Agency for Healthcare Research and Quality, Rockville, MD. 2012. Available at: http://www.ahrq.gov/professionals/clinicians-providers/guidelines-recommendations/tobacco/5steps.html. Accessed October 1, 2015.
21. Henry-Edwards S, Humeniuk R, Ali R, et al. Brief intervention for substance use: a manual for use in primary care. Geneva (Switzerland): World Health Organization; 2003.
22. Landry MJ. Overview of addiction treatment effectiveness. Pub. No. (SMA) 96–3081. Rockville (MD): Substance Abuse and Mental Health Services Administration; 1996.
23. American Psychiatric Association. Practice guidelines for treatment of patients with substance use disorders: alcohol, cocaine, opioids. Washington, DC: American Psychiatric Association; 1995.
24. Reardon C. Alternatives to 12-step addiction recovery. Social Work Today 2013; 13:12.
25. McLellan AT, Lewis DC, O'Brien CP, et al. Drug dependence, chronic medical illness implications for treatment, insurance, and outcomes evaluation. JAMA 2000;284:1689–95.
26. Sdrulla AD, Chen G. The multidisciplinary approach to the management of substance abuse. In: Substance abuse inpatient and outpatient management. New York: Springer Science+Business Media; 2015. p. 193–208.

Depression Screening, Diagnosis, and Treatment Across the Lifespan

Elizabeth W. Cozine, MD, John M. Wilkinson, MD*

KEYWORDS

- Depression • Screening • Collaborative care • Diagnosis • Treatment
- Augmentation

KEY POINTS

- Depression is common, and effective management is challenging.
- Six simple changes that all practices can implement include: empower and train office staff, develop a registry, use standardized rating instruments for diagnosis and tracking, implement stepped care and treat to target, use motivational interviewing techniques, and develop consultative relationships with mental health experts.
- Following a process of stepped care and avoiding clinical inertia by enacting proactive and timely intensification of treatment leads to better outcomes.
- Augmentation of usual depression treatment is relatively straightforward and could be more readily employed by all primary care providers.

INTRODUCTION

Depression is common,[1–3] expensive,[4–7] and shortens lives.[8] Depression contributes to the development of many chronic conditions, complicates their management, and results in poorer outcomes.[2,9]

Although evidence-based guidelines have been developed,[10–12] and effective collaborative care models have been described and implemented,[13–16] depression remains underdiagnosed and undertreated.[17]

Primary care practices will increasingly be caring for more complex patients, including those with depression and other mental health issues. Even small-to-medium sized practices, with limited resources and training, can apply the basic principles underlying collaborative care and mobilize all team members to more effectively diagnose and treat major depression. In addition, all providers, whether or not they are part of an organized system, can develop a greater familiarity and increased comfort with a wider array of treatment and augmentation strategies.

Department of Family Medicine, Mayo Clinic, 200 1st Street Southwest, Rochester, MN 55905, USA
* Corresponding author.
E-mail address: wilkinson.john@mayo.edu

Prim Care Clin Office Pract 43 (2016) 229–243
http://dx.doi.org/10.1016/j.pop.2016.02.004 **primarycare.theclinics.com**
0095-4543/16/$ – see front matter © 2016 Elsevier Inc. All rights reserved.

In recent years, other papers in *Primary Care: Clinics in Office Practice* have discussed the collaborative care model,[17] the Sequenced Treatment to Relieve Depression (STAR*D) study,[18] and depression and suicide screening strategies and tools.[19] This article focuses on 6 basic components of more effective depression care, emphasizing systems of team-based and collaborative care for diagnosis, monitoring, and follow-up. It also emphasizes the principles of stepped care and proactive and timely intensification of treatment, and discusses various augmentation strategies that all primary care providers could more readily employ.

COLLABORATIVE CARE: PRINCIPLES FOR ALL PRACTICES

Unutzer and Park listed 6 simple changes that all practices can implement to both improve care and gain valuable experience and confidence in the treatment of patients with complicated or persistent depression:

Empower and train office staff
Develop a registry
Use standardized rating instruments for diagnosis and tracking
Implement stepped care and treat to target
Use motivational interviewing techniques
Develop consultative relationships with mental health experts (**Box 1**)

These changes are within the capabilities of any primary care practice; more effective and more professionally satisfying depression care can be delivered even in the absence of a formal collaborative care system and dedicated mental health professionals.[17,20]

SCREENING

Until recently, universal screening for depression was generally conditioned upon having staff-assisted systems in place for appropriate monitoring and follow-up.[21] However, the 2016 recommendation of the US Preventive Services Task Force (USPSTF)

Box 1
Six simple changes for improved depression care

- Empower and train office personnel and support staff, in high-functioning, physician-led teams, to proactively track treatment adherence, adverse effects, and effectiveness, and to facilitate timely intensification of treatment when necessary.

- Create or utilize a registry function to enable providers and support staff to identify those patients with depression in the practice and to track their progress.

- Use a standardized, structured rating scale, such as the PHQ-9 for depression for both diagnosis and, more importantly, for tracking improvement.

- Implement stepped care and treat to target, in which all treatments are proactively modified, in a timely fashion, with remission of symptoms being the ultimate goal.

- Learn and utilize evidence-based motivational interviewing techniques in all interactions with all personnel in the practice, to enhance patient engagement and adherence.

- Seek out and develop relationships with behavioral health providers who are willing to collaborate and engage in active dialogues. particularly around more complicated and treatment-resistant patients.

Adapted from Unutzer J, Park M. Strategies to improve the management of depression in primary care. [review]. Prim Care 2012;39(2):415–31; with permission.

recognizes that support systems are "much more widely available and accepted as part of mental health care" and therefore recommends that all adults, including pregnant and postpartum women, be routinely screened in all settings.[22]

Certain groups are at greater risk for depression, including the elderly, people with a family history or prior history of mental illness, and people with chronic medical conditions. In addition, people in chaotic life situations; those who abuse drugs or alcohol; those who are widowed, divorced, or never married; and patients with multiple somatic complaints are also at increased risk.

Many of the symptoms for which patients seek help in primary care practices actually represent various manifestations of depressive illness.[23] Approximately two-thirds of patients with major depression present with somatic complaints, particularly pain, headaches, or fatigue,[24] and these patients are at greater risk of being misdiagnosed.[25]

At a minimum, practices should use a combination of clinical judgment about which patients have more somatic-type symptoms, and recognition of higher-risk patients, to target specific individuals. All team members should be alert for subtle signs and cues, whether on the phone, at front desk check-in, or when roomed by the nurse, and feel empowered to have the patient complete a screening instrument whenever it seems appropriate. Where these sorts of systems are in place, routine screening is more effective in both identifying and treating depression.[26,27]

For adolescents 12 to 18 years of age, the USPSTF continues to recommend that appropriate systems be in place before implementing universal screening, and for children younger than 12 years of age, they have concluded that there is insufficient evidence to assess the balance of benefits and harms of screening at all.[28]

Evidence-based screening recommendations and several well-validated instruments in common use are listed and discussed in greater detail in the article by Deneke and colleagues.[19]

Patient Health Questionaire-9

The Patient Health Questionaire-9 (PHQ-9) is widely used, easy to administer, and effective for assessing severity and tracking response to therapy over time. It has been validated in adults, including the elderly.[29,30]

Patient Health Questionaire-2

The PHQ-2, consisting of the first 2 questions (which ask about depressed mood and anhedonia) of the PHQ-9, is often used as an initial screen; the PHQ-9 is administered only to patients screening positive.[31]

Patient Health Questionnaire-M

The PHQ-M is modified for adolescents ages 12 to 18; it addresses increased irritability and failure to gain weight, as well as suicidality.

Edinburgh Postnatal Depression Scale

The Edinburgh Postnatal Depression Scale (EPDS) is a more sensitive screen for postpartum depression than the PHQ-9[32]; it focuses less on somatic symptoms and more on depressed mood and anhedonia.

DIAGNOSIS

For screening to be effective, it must be combined with appropriate follow-up to further evaluate the patient and to confirm or exclude a diagnosis of depression.

Screening only identifies patients at increased risk for depression; it does not make a diagnosis.[33]

A careful evaluation (and additional screening questions and tools) are still required to rule out other conditions, especially other psychiatric illnesses, including generalized anxiety disorder, bipolar disorder, alcohol and chemical dependency, or post-traumatic stress disorder.

An accurate diagnosis is also essential for ensuring appropriate follow-up and tracking; EHR registry functions require diagnostic inputs by the clinician.

Pregnant and Postpartum Women

Diagnosing postpartum depression is challenging. Women with this condition often have feelings of guilt and worthlessness, obsessive thoughts about harming their babies, and suicidal ideation. Often, they do not volunteer this information out of a sense of shame or embarrassment and must be specifically asked. Women with a personal or family history of any major depressive disorder, including postpartum depression, and those with poor social supports, are at greatest risk.

In contrast to postpartum depression, which may begin several weeks or even months after delivery and is more persistent, the baby blues begin within a few days and spontaneously resolve within 2 weeks. These women may have symptoms of crying and emotional lability, nervousness, anxiety, and sleep disturbance, but do not have thoughts of death or suicide.

To distinguish the sleep disturbance of postpartum depression from the normal disruption caused by a new baby, ask if the mother can sleep when the baby sleeps.[34]

Elderly Patients

Depression is not a natural consequence of aging, and untreated depression in the elderly may have even greater morbidity than in younger patients. Elderly men in particular have a greater rate of completed suicides than many other group. Major depressive disorder in the elderly follows Diagnostic and Statistical Manual of Mental Disorders-5 (DSM-5) criteria, although these patients may present with more subtle somatic and neurovegetative symptoms.

TREATMENT

Effective care for any chronic condition, including depression, requires ongoing monitoring and management, often including switching or adding multiple drugs, or utilizing various adjunctive therapies.

The ultimate goal of depression treatment should be remission of symptoms, rather than simply improvement. Persistent depressive symptoms (PDS), even if relatively mild, still result in significant impairments in relationships, workplace productivity, and overall health. In contrast, when remission is the endpoint, patients, providers, and team members are more fully focused on optimal stepped care and a common target for treatment.

Stepped Care and Treat to Target

All treatments must be regularly assessed for effectiveness and proactively modified in a timely fashion. Whether initially recommending medication, psychotherapy, or both, timely follow-up of all patients, beginning within a few days, to confirm that they have started treatment, and to check for adverse effects, improves treatment adherence over time.[35] Regularly assess and track improvement with the PHQ-9; this can be done by phone or secure online messaging.

Although most interventions for depression may take several weeks to reach full effectiveness, there is no advantage to waiting longer than the recommended intervals before trying a next step, whether that is a dosage increase, switching, or augmentation.

This degree of follow-up, assessment, and treatment modification is not possible without an organized system involving a trained and empowered staff, a workable registry, and the routine use of a standardized rating scale. Identify and empower interested staff members who can assist with this work. Even in highly organized, structured systems, optimal stepped care is difficult to implement. The patients themselves must be actively engaged in their treatment and progress, and in making the lifestyle changes necessary for better health.

With the support of a consulting psychiatrist, primary care providers become more experienced and more comfortable with a greater variety of medications and more intensive interventions, and derive greater satisfaction in providing the best possible evidence-based care to complex patients.[36]

Persistent depressive symptoms and clinical inertia

Patients with persistent depressive symptoms (PDS), as predicted by more complex comorbidities and higher scores on various screening instruments, consistently are more difficult to treat and require more intense interventions.[37,38]

Although failure to improve is often ascribed to treatment-resistant depression, the problem is often better explained by clinical inertia.[39] A depressive disorder should not be considered to be treatment resistant until the patient has tried maximal doses of 3 different agents for 12 weeks each and has still failed to achieve remission.[10]

Although achieving remission is difficult, even in the best of systems, clinicians must avoid giving up too soon and being satisfied with only minor degrees of improvement. Continuing to focus on the endpoint, they must shorten the time between steps, increase dosages, augment where appropriate with other agents and evidence-based psychotherapy, or switch medications.[40]

Managing expectations

Patients and providers must nonetheless have realistic expectations about the effort involved and the improvement that is likely to be achieved. These challenges and limitations should be part of an ongoing conversation as the team continues to work with each patient. Even with optimal management, many patients, particularly those with PDS and other comorbidities, may not have remission of all symptoms; however, the outcomes are generally better than those with usual care and are worth the effort.

First Steps, Shared Decision Making, and Patient Engagement

Very often, the initial discussion with the patient revolves around whether the patient is depressed and the necessity of doing something other than the status quo.[41] This negotiation requires tact, patience, and sensitivity.[42] Once the provider is confident of the diagnosis, try to overcome early clinical inertia by mutually agreeing to do something, even if it is simply a commitment to further follow-up or a return visit within a specific period of time. It is often helpful to engage other team members at the beginning, introducing them with a warm handoff. Taking these first steps can be a significant confidence builder for patients.[43]

For minor or subsyndromal depression, there is no evidence psychotherapy or antidepressants provide significant benefit. However, follow-up is warranted to provide timely intervention in the event that symptoms progress to a major depressive episode.

For mild-to-moderate depression, psychotherapy and pharmacotherapy are equally effective, but of limited benefit; STAR*D patients clearly preferred starting with medications. However, psychotherapy may decrease the frequency and severity of recurrences.[44,45]

For more severe depression, a combination of psychotherapy and pharmacotherapy is more effective than either one alone.

Among the second-generation antidepressants, all agents are equally effective; any of the selective serotonin reuptake inhibitors (SSRIs), fluoxetine, paroxetine, citalopram, or sertraline, are a good first step (**Table 1**).[11] Bupropion, with a different mechanism of action, is also an effective antidepressant and a reasonable choice as an initial therapy. Although bupropion does not cause sexual dysfunction or weight gain, it is somewhat more activating and can lower the seizure threshold. If patients can recall what medications have worked for them in the past or find out which have been effective in their relatives, consider using this information as a basis for initial treatment.

Discuss the expected length of treatment. Many patients are particularly concerned that even starting an antidepressant commits them to taking medication indefinitely, although in real-world clinical practice, stopping too early is far more common. In general, advise treating the first episode of major depression for 6 to 12 months and the second episode for 12 to 24 months; however, after 3 recurrences, encourage the patient to consider long-term treatment.

Of perhaps greater relevance, patients should know that there is a high likelihood that they will eventually require additional or alternate therapy, as only 30% achieve meaningful improvement on the first therapy, and only two-thirds of those patients sustain that improvement.

Discuss expectations of adverse effects and provide reassurance. All psychoactive medications will cause some adverse effects in most patients. Fortunately, if the starting dose is low, and changes are made slowly, most symptoms will resolve. If patients know what to expect and are proactively contacted by office staff for timely reassurance, this is often all that is needed to keep the patient from stopping treatment prematurely.

With most antidepressants, it takes 3 to 4 weeks to achieve the full benefit of any dose; if there is no significant improvement after that time, increase the dose. However, if the patient seems to be improving, it is reasonable to wait for up to 8 to 12 weeks, while continuing to maintain contact, before making any changes.

Adolescents and young adults
There is an FDA black box warning regarding suicide risk in adolescents and young adults taking SSRIs. This is based on the observation that these patients had more suicidal ideation and thoughts of death during the early stages of treatment. It is important to share with adolescents and their parents that there were not more completed suicides or even attempts, and the risks associated with depression left untreated are far greater. Nonetheless, close follow-up is mandatory. Fluoxetine is generally well tolerated, is among the best-studied antidepressants in adolescents, is FDA-approved for use in adolescents, and is an excellent first-line treatment.

Pregnant and postpartum women
There are conflicting data on the risk of birth defects in the babies born to women who take antidepressants during pregnancy. Although all studies have some limitations, the most recent (and most thorough) study to date found that citalopram, escitalopram, and sertraline do not seem to cause any problems, although there may be a

Table 1
Second-generation antidepressants

Classification	Key Points	Typical Daily Dose
Selective serotonin reuptake inhibitors (SSRIs)		
Citalopram (Celexa)	May cause QT prolongation, especially at higher doses (>40 mg)	20–40 mg
Escitalopram (Lexapro)	May have faster onset than citalopram More likely to cause weight gain QT prolongation less likely than with citalopram	10–20 mg
Fluoxetine (Prozac)	May cause overstimulation or agitation in elderly	20–60 mg
Paroxetine (Paxil)	Short half-life: more discontinuation symptoms Anticholinergic effects (especially in elderly) More likely to cause sexual dysfunction More likely to cause weight gain	20–40 mg
Sertraline (Zoloft)	May cause more diarrhea	50–150 mg
Serotonin-norepinephrine reuptake inhibitors (SNRIs)		
Desvenlafaxine, extended-release (Pristiq)	Short half-life: more discontinuation symptoms May cause more nausea and vomiting	50 mg
Venlafaxine, immediate-release (Effexor)	Short half-life, more discontinuation symptoms May cause more nausea and vomiting	75–375 mg (must be divided into BID dosing)
Venlafaxine, extended-release (Effexor XR)	Longer half-life and less discontinuation symptoms (than immediate-release venlafaxine) May be dosed once daily May cause more nausea and vomiting	75–225 mg
Mirtazapine (Remeron)	Faster onset (2 wk) Significant long-term weight gain Increased somnolence	15–45 mg
Duloxetine (Cymbalta)	Has FDA indication for chronic pain, but trials are equivocal	30–120 mg
Dopamine–norepinephrine reuptake inhibitors		
Bupropion, sustained-release (Wellbutrin SR)	Often used as adjunct Few sexual side effects Avoid in patients with anxiety Slight risk of seizure	300–400 mg (must be divided into twice daily dosing)
Bupropion, extended-release (Wellbutrin XL)	Often used as adjunct Few sexual side effects Avoid in patients with anxiety Slight risk of seizure	150–450 mg
Serotonin antagonist and reuptake inhibitors: serotonin modulators (SARI)		
Trazodone	Increased somnolence Typically used at bedtime as adjunct for residual insomnia	50–150 mg

Data from Refs.[10–12]

very low absolute increase in cardiac and pulmonary abnormalities with paroxetine and fluoxetine.[46] In absolute terms, the incidence increases from an approximate baseline of 1 in 1000 births to 2 in 1000 births. This is much lower than the risks associated with either smoking or alcohol use during pregnancy, or the risks associated with untreated depression.

All second-generation antidepressants seem to be safe for breastfeeding babies; there is no consistent evidence of any clinically significant symptoms in these infants.

Elderly patients
In general, the SSRIs and other second-generation antidepressants are well tolerated in the elderly; however, because of concerns about adverse effects, the starting dose should be one-half of the doses used in younger individuals, and increases should be made more slowly. However, dosages should still be increased as tolerated until the desired benefit is achieved.

Mirtazapine for agitation and anorexia in the elderly Mirtazapine, with both a sedating and appetite-stimulating effect, is particularly useful for elderly patients whose depression is complicated by insomnia and loss of appetite.

Do not use tricyclic antidepressants (TCAs) in the elderly because of their increased anticholinergic adverse effects, particularly urinary retention and syncope, as well as their potential to unmask occult cardiac conduction abnormalities.[47,48]

Patients with cognitive impairment
Depression is common in patients with mild cognitive impairment. The SSRIs are well tolerated in this group, not infrequently resulting in a surprising improvement in function.

Patients who use tobacco
For smokers with major depression, bupropion and nortriptyline should be considered, as they increase cessation rates by about twofold.[12]

Patients with alcohol abuse and chemical dependency
Alcohol use, even if not at the level of alcohol abuse, as well as other types of chemical dependency, complicates the treatment of depression. However, continued alcohol use should not be seen as a rationale to forgo treatment. SSRIs and TCAs are well tolerated, even in the face of heavy alcohol use. As bupropion can lower the seizure threshold, consider other agents in patients who may be at risk for alcohol or benzodiazepine withdrawal.

Early Challenges: Close Follow-up and Patient Activation
Utilizing the registry, continue to maintain regular, close contact on a weekly basis or so; address side effects, counsel patience, and track patients' progress with the PHQ-9.[49]

At this point, the goal is to help people avoid giving up too early[50] and to begin to move to greater engagement, wherein activated patients take responsibility for self-care, including engaging in pleasurable activities, practicing mindfulness,[51] getting regular exercise,[52–54] and assessing and monitoring their own progress.

Motivational interviewing and patient activation
All members of the team who interact with these patients can become familiar with principles of motivational interviewing; they can learn and utilize evidence-based motivational interviewing techniques in all interactions to enhance patient engagement and adherence.[17]

Try Something Else: Switching, Augmentation, or Both?

After 8 to 12 weeks of treatment at optimal doses, if patients have not achieved remission of their symptoms, the provider should work with them to try something else. First of all, reconsider the diagnosis; in particular, assess again for alcohol or other chemical dependency, comorbid anxiety, PTSD, or bipolar depression.

In general, if there has been no response to the initial therapy, consider switching to another monotherapy as the next step.[55] If there has been a partial response, consider augmentation of the first medication with a second.[56]

Commonly used second monotherapies are sertraline, extended-release bupropion, and extended-release venlafaxine. Extended-release bupropion is also commonly used for augmentation, as is buspirone or cognitive behavioral therapy (CBT). The augmentation strategy chosen is best dictated by the specific ongoing or residual symptoms or adverse effects. In STAR*D, patients who were intolerant to 1 SSRI (citalopram) did not have any more likelihood of intolerance to another (sertraline).

Frequently patients will have already discontinued treatment on their own, and there is actually very little specific information to guide the clinician in switching among antidepressants. If switching from 1 SSRI to another, or from 1 serotonin-norepinephrine reuptake inhibitor (SNRI) to another, it seems reasonable to completely taper off of the first agent before starting the second. However, when switching from an SSRI to an SNRI or vice versa, the second agent could be initiated at a low dose while still tapering the first. Fluoxetine, because of its extremely long half-life, is the 1 exception; it should be allowed to wash out completely for a week or so before starting any other medication.

If there is no significant improvement on two consecutive monotherapies, very little is likely to be gained by switching again. At this point, formal psychiatric consultation is reasonable, although more informal "curbside consultations" are also helpful, particularly for advice about augmentation strategies.[57]

Serotonin Syndrome: Increasingly Common with More Intense Treatments

Serotonin syndrome, often the result of combining multiple serotonergic medications, is increasingly common but still relatively unfamiliar to many clinicians. While the second-generation antidepressants are generally safer than the older agents, the trend toward higher doses and augmentation strategies may still increase the risk.

In addition, clinicians may not recognize that many common medications, prescribed for other indications, may also have serotoninergic effects. In particular, the pain relievers tramadol and fentanyl, the muscle relaxant cyclobenzaprine, the antiemetics metoclopramide and ondansetron, the cough preparation dextromethorphan, as well as the amphetamine stimulants and various antimigraine drugs, when taken by patients already on antidepressants, may precipitate this syndrome.

Clinicians should become familiar with the serotonin syndrome and not ignore more subtle and nonspecific symptoms in patients on antidepressants. If recognized, these may be valuable, early clues that a more serious, life-threatening condition might be precipitated if another serotoninergic agent is added. Serotonin syndrome, or the potential for its development, should be suspected in any patient showing mental status changes (agitation, restlessness, anxiety, confusion), neuromuscular hyperactivity (rigidity, hypertonia, clonus, teeth clenching), or autonomic instability (tachycardia, tachypnea, fever, diarrhea, sweating, flushing). Most cases are relatively mild; stopping the offending medications usually results in symptom resolution.[58,59]

Augmentation Strategies for Specific Symptoms

The most common augmentation strategies in STAR*D were adding extended-release bupropion, buspirone, or CBT to the initial monotherapy.[18] The augmentation strategy chosen is best dictated by the specific ongoing or residual symptoms.

Bupropion augmentation for sexual dysfunction or persistent fatigue

For patients who have had a partial response, bupropion is an effective second agent.[56] The addition of bupropion may also alleviate sexual side effects, or correct persistent lassitude.

Serotonin-norepinephrine reuptake inhibitor or TCA augmentation for chronic pain complicating depression

Consider a TCA (amitriptyline, nortriptyline) or an SNRI (duloxetine has an FDA indication for treating chronic pain).

Trazodone or mirtazapine augmentation for persistent sleep disturbance

Trazodone, a serotonin antagonist and reuptake inhibitor (SARI), is an older second-generation antidepressant. It shares some properties with the SSRIs; and while safer and with fewer anticholinergic side effects than the TCAs,[60] sedation and orthostatic hypotension, especially in the elderly, generally still preclude its use at full therapeutic doses. Rather, prescribe trazodone 50 to 150 mg at bedtime as an adjunct to other agents. At these doses, the risk of serotonin syndrome is minimal.[61]

Mirtazapine, 15 to 30 mg at bedtime, while often effective, is limited by its potential for causing significant appetite stimulation and weight gain.

Thyroid augmentation for persistent fatigue and vegetative symptoms

Thyroid augmentation with either liothyronine (T3) (25–50 μg once daily) or levothyroxine (T4) (15–50 μg once daily) is often effective, although few good quality studies have been done (particularly with SSRIs); observed benefits may be due to the correction of subclinical hypothyroidism. Patients who respond will do so within 1 to 2 weeks; if there is no response after 3 weeks, discontinue treatment.[62] At such low doses, even with long-term use, thyroid suppression is unlikely; however, occasional thyroid-stimulating hormone (TSH) testing is reasonable.[63]

Lithium augmentation for mood stabilization

For patients who do not meet criteria for bipolar disorder but who are experiencing manic-type symptoms, lithium augmentation is an option. Again, most studies that have been done are older and with TCAs; there are few with SSRIs. The usual dose is 450 to 900 mg per day. Monitor both renal and thyroid function; check creatinine at baseline and every 12 months and TSH at baseline and every 6 months. In addition, monitor lithium levels periodically; the target range is 0.4 to 0.08 mmol/L, although serum levels may only partially correlate with response. In spite of potential drug–drug issues, particularly with nonsteroidal anti-inflammatory drugs (NSAIDs), diuretics, and other psychotropic medications, lithium augmentation is a potentially helpful strategy for patients who are struggling and need something to stabilize their mood until they can see a psychiatrist.[62,64,65]

Buspirone augmentation for persistent anxiety

For patients on maximal doses of antidepressants who are still anxious, buspirone augmentation is often effective; it has no anticonvulsant or muscle relaxant properties and is nonaddictive. After advancing to optimal doses, it may take more than 2 weeks to see its anxiolytic effect. The starting dose is 5 mg twice daily; advance to 10 mg twice daily after 1 week and to 15 mg twice daily after 2 weeks. A dose as high as

30 mg twice daily may be required. Buspirone may also be helpful in other clinical settings, including PDS[56] or to reverse SSRI-induced bruxism or sexual dysfunction.[66]

Bright light therapy for seasonal depression
A light box is often useful as an adjunct to medication for major depression complicated by seasonal variation, or used alone for milder seasonal depressive symptoms. Patients with more atypical mood symptoms—increased appetite and increased sleeping—may respond best. The dose is bright light of 10,000 lux for 30 to 60 minutes every morning.[53]

Hold the Gains: Prevention and Treatment of Relapse

Continue treatment even after relapse has been achieved, and continue to stay in contact with the patient.[67] To reiterate, advise treating the first episode of major depression for 6 to 12 months and the second episode for 12 to 24 months; however, after 3 recurrences, encourage the patient to consider long-term treatment.

If remission has been maintained for 1 to 2 years, and the patient wishes to try discontinuing treatment, taper the medication slowly. A general approach would be to decrease the dose by 25% to 50% every 1 to 2 weeks or even longer, over several weeks or even months. For drugs with shorter half-lives, particularly venlafaxine and paroxetine, consider tapering by even smaller increments, over a longer period of time.

Selective serotonin reuptake inhibitor discontinuation syndrome
In addition to symptoms in common with major depression (dysphoria, appetite and sleep disturbances, fatigue, and difficulty concentrating), patients with SSRI discontinuation syndrome may also experience dizziness, electric shock sensations, sensations in the face and extremities, rushing sensations in the head, headache, and nausea. These symptoms will resolve within a few days of restarting the medication.[68]

SUMMARY

Effective management of patients suffering from depression is difficult work; under the best of circumstances, patients may not respond to treatment, much less achieve a sustained remission. In the authors' experience, primary care providers, as well as their teams, have found that working within a collaborative care model is an iterative process. As they work together, and develop supportive relationships with one another and with consultants, they become more comfortable with increasingly complex patients and their abilities to guide patients on what, for many, is a life-long journey.

REFERENCES

1. Kessler RC, Chiu WT, Demler O, et al. Prevalence, severity, and comorbidity of 12-month DSM-IV disorders in the National Comorbidity Survey Replication. Arch Gen Psychiatry 2005;62(6):617–27.
2. Strine TW, Mokdad AH, Balluz LS, et al. Depression and anxiety in the United States: findings from the 2006 behavioral risk factor surveillance system. Psychiatr Serv 2008;59(12):1383–90.
3. Centers for Disease Control and Prevention (CDC). Current depression among adults—United States, 2006 and 2008. MMWR Morb Mortal Wkly Rep 2010; 59(38):1229–35.
4. Beck A, Crain AL, Solberg LI, et al. Severity of depression and magnitude of productivity loss. Ann Fam Med 2011;9(4):305–11.

5. Unutzer J, Patrick DL, Simon G, et al. Depressive symptoms and the cost of health services in HMO patients aged 65 years and older. A 4-year prospective study. JAMA 1997;277(20):1618–23.

6. Katon WJ, Lin E, Russo J, et al. Increased medical costs of a population-based sample of depressed elderly patients. Arch Gen Psychiatry 2003;60(9):897–903.

7. Greenberg PE, Fournier AA, Sisitsky T, et al. The economic burden of adults with major depressive disorder in the United States (2005 and 2010). J Clin Psychiatry 2015;76(2):155–62.

8. Cuijpers P, Smit F. Excess mortality in depression: a meta-analysis of community studies. J Affect Disord 2002;72(3):227–36.

9. Katon WJ. Clinical and health services relationships between major depression, depressive symptoms, and general medical illness. Biol Psychiatry 2003;54(3):216–26.

10. Mitchell J, Trangle M, Degnan B, et al. Institute for Clinical Systems Improvement. Adult Depression in Primary Care. 2013. Available at: https://www.icsi.org/guidelines__more/catalog_guidelines_and_more/catalog_guidelines/catalog_behavioral_health_guidelines/depression/. Accessed March 6, 2016.

11. Qaseem A, Snow V, Denberg TD, et al. Using second-generation antidepressants to treat depressive disorders: a clinical practice guideline from the American College of Physicians. Ann Intern Med 2008;149(10):725–33.

12. Gelenberg AJ, Freeman MP, Markowitz JC, et al. American Psychiatric Association. Practice guideline for the treatment of patients with major depressive disorder. 2010. Available at: http://psychiatryonline.org/pb/assets/raw/sitewide/practice_guidelines/guidelines/mdd.pdf. Accessed July 31, 2015.

13. Katon W, Von Korff M, Lin E, et al. Stepped collaborative care for primary care patients with persistent symptoms of depression: a randomized trial. Arch Gen Psychiatry 1999;56(12):1109–15.

14. Katon WJ, Seelig M. Population-based care of depression: team care approaches to improving outcomes. J Occup Environ Med 2008;50(4):459–67.

15. Gilbody S, Bower P, Fletcher J, et al. Collaborative care for depression: a cumulative meta-analysis and review of longer-term outcomes. Arch Intern Med 2006;166(21):2314–21.

16. Unutzer J, Katon W, Callahan CM, et al. Collaborative care management of late-life depression in the primary care setting: a randomized controlled trial. JAMA 2002;288(22):2836–45.

17. Unutzer J, Park M. Strategies to improve the management of depression in primary care. Prim Care Clin Office Pract 2012;39(2):415–31.

18. Cain RA. Navigating the Sequenced Treatment Alternatives to Relieve Depression (STAR*D) study: practical outcomes and implications for depression treatment in primary care. Prim Care Clin Office Pract 2007;34(3):505–19, vi.

19. Deneke DE, Schultz H, Fluent TE. Screening for depression in the primary care population. Prim Care Clin Office Pract 2014;41(2):399–420.

20. Hunkeler EM, Meresman JF, Hargreaves WA, et al. Efficacy of nurse telehealth care and peer support in augmenting treatment of depression in primary care. Arch Fam Med 2000;9(8):700–8.

21. U.S. Preventive Services. Screening for depression in adults: U.S. Preventive Services Task Force Recommendation Statement. Ann Intern Med 2009;151:784–92.

22. Siu AL, U.S. Preventive Services Task Force (USPSTF). Screening for depression in adults: U.S. Preventive Services Task Force Recommendation Statement. JAMA 2016;315(4):380–7.

23. Henningsen P, Zimmermann T, Sattel H. Medically unexplained physical symptoms, anxiety, and depression: a meta-analytic review. Psychosom Med 2003; 65(4):528–33.
24. Tylee A, Gandhi P. The importance of somatic symptoms in depression in primary care. Prim Care Companion J Clin Psychiatry 2005;7(4):167–76.
25. Timonen M, Liukkonen T. Management of depression in adults. BMJ 2008; 336(7641):435–9.
26. O'Connor EA, Whitlock EP, Gaynes B, et al. Screening for depression in adults and older adults in primary care: an updated systematic review. Evidence Synthesis No. 75. AHRQ Publication No. 10-05143-EF-1. Rockville, Maryland: Agency for Healthcare Research and Quality, December 2009.
27. Pignone M, Gaynes BN, Rushton JL, et al. Screening for Depression. Systematic Evidence Review No. 6. AHRQ Publication No. 02-S002. Rockville, MD: Agency for Healthcare Research and Quality; 2002.
28. Siu AL, U.S. Preventive Services Task Force (USPSTF). Screening for depression in children and adolescents: U.S. Preventive Services Task Force Recommendation Statement. Ann Intern Med 2016;164:360–6.
29. Kroenke K, Spitzer RL, Williams JB. The PHQ-9: validity of a brief depression severity measure. J Gen Intern Med 2001;16(9):606–13.
30. Kroenke K, Spitzer RL, Williams JB, et al. The patient health questionnaire somatic, anxiety, and depressive symptom scales: a systematic review. Gen Hosp Psychiatry 2010;32(4):345–59.
31. Kroenke K, Spitzer RL, Williams JB. The patient health questionnaire-2: validity of a two-item depression screener. Med Care 2003;41(11):1284–92.
32. Hanusa BH, Scholle SH, Haskett RF, et al. Screening for depression in the postpartum period: a comparison of three instruments. J Womens Health (Larchmt) 2008;17(4):585–96.
33. American Psychiatric Association. American Psychiatric Association DSM-5 task force. diagnostic and statistical manual of mental disorders: DSM-5. 5th edition. Washington, DC: American Psychiatric Association; 2013.
34. Hirst KP, Moutier CY. Postpartum major depression. Am Fam Physician 2010; 82(8):926–33.
35. Bull SA, Hu XH, Hunkeler EM, et al. Discontinuation of use and switching of antidepressants: influence of patient-physician communication. JAMA 2002; 288(11):1403–9.
36. Levine S, Unutzer J, Yip JY, et al. Physicians' satisfaction with a collaborative disease management program for late-life depression in primary care. Gen Hosp Psychiatry 2005;27(6):383–91.
37. Angstman KB, Shippee ND, Maclaughlin KL, et al. Patient self-assessment factors predictive of persistent depressive symptoms 6 months after enrollment in collaborative care management. Depress Anxiety 2013;30(2):143–8.
38. Angstman KB, Pietruszewski P, Rasmussen NH, et al. Depression remission after six months of collaborative care management: role of initial severity of depression in outcome. Ment Health Fam Med 2012;9(2):99–106.
39. Henke RM, Zaslavsky AM, McGuire TG, et al. Clinical inertia in depression treatment. Med Care 2009;47(9):959–67.
40. Keller MB. Issues in treatment-resistant depression. J Clin Psychiatry 2005; 66(Suppl 8):5–12.
41. Baik SY, Gonzales JJ, Bowers BJ, et al. Reinvention of depression instruments by primary care clinicians. Ann Fam Med 2010;8(3):224–30.

42. Hunot VM, Horne R, Leese MN, et al. A cohort study of adherence to antidepressants in primary care: the influence of antidepressant concerns and treatment preferences. Prim Care Companion J Clin Psychiatry 2007;9(2):91–9.

43. Garfield S, Francis SA, Smith FJ. Building concordant relationships with patients starting antidepressant medication. Patient Educ Couns 2004;55(2):241–6.

44. Hollon SD, Jarrett RB, Nierenberg AA, et al. Psychotherapy and medication in the treatment of adult and geriatric depression: which monotherapy or combined treatment? J Clin Psychiatry 2005;66(4):455–68.

45. Hollon SD, DeRubeis RJ, Shelton RC, et al. Prevention of relapse following cognitive therapy vs medications in moderate to severe depression. Arch Gen Psychiatry 2005;62(4):417–22.

46. Reefhuis J, Devine O, Friedman JM, et al. Specific SSRIs and birth defects: bayesian analysis to interpret new data in the context of previous reports. BMJ 2015;351:h3190.

47. Birrer RB, Vemuri SP. Depression in later life: a diagnostic and therapeutic challenge. Am Fam Physician 2004;69(10):2375–82.

48. Gasto C, Navarro V, Marcos T, et al. Single-blind comparison of venlafaxine and nortriptyline in elderly major depression. J Clin Psychopharmacol 2003;23(1): 21–6.

49. Lowe B, Unutzer J, Callahan CM, et al. Monitoring depression treatment outcomes with the patient health questionnaire-9. Med Care 2004;42(12):1194–201.

50. Lin EH, Von Korff M, Ludman EJ, et al. Enhancing adherence to prevent depression relapse in primary care. Gen Hosp Psychiatry 2003;25(5):303–10.

51. Klainin-Yobas P, Cho MA, Creedy D. Efficacy of mindfulness-based interventions on depressive symptoms among people with mental disorders: a meta-analysis. Int J Nurs Stud 2012;49(1):109–21.

52. Dunn AL, Trivedi MH, Kampert JB, et al. Exercise treatment for depression: efficacy and dose response. Am J Prev Med 2005;28(1):1–8.

53. Leppamaki SJ, Partonen TT, Hurme J, et al. Randomized trial of the efficacy of bright-light exposure and aerobic exercise on depressive symptoms and serum lipids. J Clin Psychiatry 2002;63(4):316–21.

54. Saeed SA, Antonacci DJ, Bloch RM. Exercise, yoga, and meditation for depressive and anxiety disorders. Am Fam Physician 2010;81(8):981–6.

55. Rush AJ, Trivedi MH, Wisniewski SR, et al. Bupropion-SR, sertraline, or venlafaxine-XR after failure of SSRIs for depression. N Engl J Med 2006; 354(12):1231–42.

56. Trivedi MH, Fava M, Wisniewski SR, et al. Medication augmentation after the failure of SSRIs for depression. N Engl J Med 2006;354(12):1243–52.

57. Cook DA, Sorensen KJ, Wilkinson JM. Value and process of curbside consultations in clinical practice: a grounded theory study. Mayo Clin Proc 2014;89(5): 602–14.

58. Boyer EW, Shannon M. The serotonin syndrome. N Engl J Med 2005;352(11): 1112–20.

59. Iqbal MM, Basil MJ, Kaplan J, et al. Overview of serotonin syndrome. Ann Clin Psychiatry 2012;24(4):310–8.

60. Rakel RE. The greater safety of trazodone over tricyclic antidepressant agents: 5-year experience in the United States. Psychopathology 1987;20(Suppl 1): 57–63.

61. Stahl SM. Stahl's essential psychopharmacology: neuroscientific basis and practical application. 4th edition. Cambridge (United Kingdom): Cambridge University Press; 2013.

62. Nierenberg AA, Fava M, Trivedi MH, et al. A comparison of lithium and T(3) augmentation following two failed medication treatments for depression: a STAR*D report. Am J Psychiatry 2006;163(9):1519–30 [quiz: 1665].
63. Pecina J, Garrison GM, Bernard ME. Levothyroxine dosage is associated with stability of thyroid-stimulating hormone values. Am J Med 2014;127(3):240–5.
64. Joffe RT, Singer W, Levitt AJ, et al. A placebo-controlled comparison of lithium and triiodothyronine augmentation of tricyclic antidepressants in unipolar refractory depression. Arch Gen Psychiatry 1993;50(5):387–93.
65. Katona CL, Abou-Saleh MT, Harrison DA, et al. Placebo-controlled trial of lithium augmentation of fluoxetine and lofepramine. Br J Psychiatry 1995;166(1):80–6.
66. Dimitriou EC, Dimitriou CE. Buspirone augmentation of antidepressant therapy. J Clin Psychopharmacol 1998;18(6):465–9.
67. Kim KH, Lee SM, Paik JW, et al. The effects of continuous antidepressant treatment during the first 6 months on relapse or recurrence of depression. J Affect Disord 2011;132(1–2):121–9.
68. Geddes JR, Carney SM, Davies C, et al. Relapse prevention with antidepressant drug treatment in depressive disorders: a systematic review. Lancet 2003; 361(9358):653–61.

Anxiety Disorders in Primary Care

Danielle H. Metzler, MD[a], David Mahoney, MD, MBE[b], John R. Freedy, MD, PhD[a],*

KEYWORDS

- Anxiety disorders • Primary care • Generalized anxiety disorder
- Social anxiety disorder • Panic disorder • Pharmacologic treatment
- Collaborative care

KEY POINTS

- Anxiety disorders are highly prevalent, with an estimated lifetime prevalence of 29% in the United States.
- Screening all patients for anxiety is not currently recommended. However, when suspected, a useful screening tool is the Generalized Anxiety Disorder scale–2, which asks 2 questions and is approximately 86% sensitive for detecting generalized anxiety disorder.
- Selective serotonin reuptake inhibitors and serotonin-norepinephrine reuptake inhibitors are first-line treatment options for anxiety. Tricyclic antidepressants are effective but, given their risky side-effect profile, are now considered third-line agents. Benzodiazepines are also effective, but because of their risk for dependence, providers should prescribe with caution and ideally for time-limited periods (days to weeks).
- Psychotherapy is found to be as effective as pharmacotherapy in the treatment of most anxiety disorders and for best results should be used in conjunction with medication.
- An emerging model for managing mental health problems in primary care settings is the collaborative care model. This model shows great promise and likely will become a sustainable approach to many mental health issues addressed in primary care settings.

INTRODUCTION

Anxiety disorders are the most common mental health disorders evaluated and treated in a primary care setting.[1] Lifetime prevalence is as high as 29% in the United States.[2] Patients suffering from anxiety disorders experience lower quality of life,[3] decreased productivity, and increased rates of medical services use. Kroenke and colleagues[1] found that those with anxiety disorders had a higher rate of self-reported disability

[a] Trident Family Medicine Residency, Department of Family Medicine, Medical University of South Carolina, 9228 Medical Plaza Drive, Charleston, SC 29406, USA; [b] Mount Pleasant Family Practice, Roper St. Francis Physicians, 1400 Hospital Dr., Mount Pleasant, South Carolina, 29464, USA
* Corresponding author.
E-mail address: freedyjr@musc.edu

Prim Care Clin Office Pract 43 (2016) 245–261
http://dx.doi.org/10.1016/j.pop.2016.02.002   **primarycare.theclinics.com**
0095-4543/16/$ – see front matter © 2016 Elsevier Inc. All rights reserved.

days (11.2–30.6) compared with those with no anxiety disorder (5.7). Further, anxiety disorders cause a significant economic burden and have become an escalating public health dilemma.

As the health care system evolves and proceeds toward a more comprehensive and integrative approach to patient care, primary care physicians must be able to recognize and initiate treatment of anxiety disorders. Interestingly, anxiety disorders are regularly misdiagnosed by primary care providers, often because the patient presents with somatic complaints.[4,5] In fact, estimates are that less than a quarter of patients present with feelings of anxiety as the chief complaint and that almost half of patients actually present with a somatic complaint.[4] Rates of misdiagnosis in one study were as high as 71% for generalized anxiety disorder (GAD).[4] In addition, many patients experience subthreshold symptoms and, as expected, contribute to the vast population of missed diagnoses and overlooked opportunities for treatment.[4]

Patients with psychiatric disorders tend to incur more visits with health care providers. Thus, prevalence data should be interpreted with caution, as it is often collected from clinic populations in which the sample of patients with psychiatric disorders is higher than that of the general population.[6]

SCREENING

Despite the widespread prevalence of anxiety disorders in primary care, there are no concrete data suggesting a benefit to screening.[6] There are no current United States Preventive Services Task Force recommendations on screening for anxiety disorders. However, there are several tools that can be used in a primary care office to screen for anxiety when the diagnosis is suspected. The Generalized Anxiety Disorder-7 (GAD-7) is the most well-known and has been validated for GAD, as well as for panic disorder and posttraumatic stress disorder (PTSD).[6] Recently, an abbreviated version, the GAD-2, has been shown to be 86% sensitive and 83% specific for detecting GAD when a score of 3 or more is tallied.[1] Composed of the first 2 questions of the GAD-7, the GAD-2 asks, "over the last 2 weeks, how often have you been bothered by the following problems: (a) feeling nervous, anxious or on edge, and (b) not being able to stop or control worrying?"[1] (**Table 1**).

The Beck Anxiety Inventory is a screening tool that helps distinguish between anxiety disorders and depressive disorders.[6] It is a 21-item questionnaire that is often used in outpatient psychiatric clinics.[6] A truncated version has been developed and tailored for primary care use—the Beck Anxiety Inventory–Primary Care—but has not yet been widely adapted.[6]

A multistage screening tool called *The Symptom Driven Diagnostic System–Primary Care* is a 16-item patient survey that screens for multiple mental health disorders in a primary care setting.[7] The pilot study found a 90% sensitivity and only 54% specificity in detecting generalized anxiety disorder.[7] Sensitivity was even lower for panic disorder at roughly 78%.[7] The advantage to this screening tool is that it is patient administered, saving the primary care provider time. In addition, this tool attempts to screen for several psychiatric disorders, helping to point the clinician in the right direction. However, it is not readily available, and the true efficacy in real-world practice is currently unknown.[6]

Several PTSD screening tests have been used in both military and civilian primary care settings. The most brief of these screening tests is the 4-item Primary Care PTSD Screen. Four yes/no questions are keyed to possible PTSD symptoms occurring within the past month: nightmares/intrusive thoughts, thought/situational avoidance, hypervigilance/easily startle, and numb/detached feeling.[8] Freedy and colleagues[9]

Table 1
Generalized anxiety disorder-7 (Generalized anxiety disorder-2)

Over the Last 2 wk, How Often Have You Been Bothered by the Following Problems?	Not at All	Several Days	More than Half the Days	Nearly Every Day
1. Feeling nervous, anxious or on edge	0	1	2	3
2. Not being able to stop or control worrying	0	1	2	3
3. Worrying too much about different things	0	1	2	3
4. Trouble relaxing	0	1	2	3
5. Being so restless that it is hard to sit still	0	1	2	3
6. Becoming easily annoyed or irritable	0	1	2	3
7. Feeling afraid as if something awful might happen	0	1	2	3
Total score:				
If you checked off any problems, how difficult have these problems made it for you to do your work, take care of things at home, or get along with other people?	Not difficult at all	Somewhat difficult	Very difficult	Extremely difficult

Bold indicates questions used in the GAD-2.
A GAD-2 score of 3 or more has an 86% sensitivity and an 83% specificity for detecting GAD.[1]
A GAD-7 score of 10 or more has an 89% sensitivity and an 82% specificity for detecting GAD.[44]
GAD-7 scores of 5, 10, and 15 may be represent mild, moderate and severe levels of anxiety, respectively.[44]
From Spitzer RL, Kroenke K, Williams JB, et al; A brief measure for assessing generalized anxiety disorder: the GAD-7. Arch Intern Med 2006;166(10):1092–7.
GAD-7 © Pfizer Inc. all rights reserved.

used a civilian primary care sample to determine a sensitivity of 85.1% and a specificity of 82.0% based on a cutoff score of 3, using the Clinician-Administered PTSD Scale as the gold standard comparison. Similar sensitivity and specificity figures have been found for military samples.[8]

Although screening for anxiety disorders is not routinely recommended for every patient, it may still be beneficial, particularly if there are systems in place to care for the patients who screen positive. Primary care providers who have a good working relationship with mental health professionals in the community can help these patients navigate their way through the medical system to a more comprehensive care plan for their mental health.

INITIAL EVALUATION

Most (70%–90%) patients with anxiety or depression present to their primary care provider with a somatic complaint.[10] Some may report one specific, distressing symptom (eg, diarrhea or insomnia), whereas others may complain of a variety of seemingly unrelated symptoms.[11] Headaches, gastrointestinal disturbances, muscle tension, chest pain or tightness, and palpitations are common physical symptoms experienced by patients with anxiety. Symptoms unable to be medically explained after an initial workup should raise the clinician's suspicion of an anxiety or depressive disorder.[12] Approximately 40% to 50% of patients with medically unexplained symptoms have an anxiety disorder, regardless of the specific symptom(s).[13] Although the nature of the physical complaints does not, the number of somatic symptoms does seem to correlate with a higher probability of an underlying psychiatric disorder.[13]

While the diagnosis of a mental health disorder is being considered, the provider should carefully consider possible medical causes for the patient's complaints. In this context, it is imperative that the provider remain empathic and encouraging toward the patient. All patients (and most especially anxious patients) wish to be heard and have their concerns taken seriously. In so doing, the provider invests in a trusting and constructive doctor-patient relationship that will eventually become the basis for accepting the diagnosis (whether a mental or physical health issue, or both) and recommended management plan. Premature reassurance can be counterproductive with anxious patients who may feel misunderstood and disrespected if not approached in a thoughtful and methodical manner. A thorough workup may be required in some patients before the diagnosis of anxiety will be accepted. Medical causes of anxiety that are most widely reported tend to be endocrine or neurologic in etiology.[14] Basic laboratory work may be warranted, such as a metabolic panel, thyroid function tests, or cortisol levels, to rule out electrolyte abnormalities, hyperthyroidism, or Cushing syndrome, respectively. Careful inquiry into the patient's medical and social history should include questions regarding use of medications, illicit substances, vitamins, or herbs. Caffeine and alcohol intake, as well as nicotine use, should be quantified.[11]

GENERALIZED ANXIETY DISORDER

The lifetime prevalence of GAD has been reported to range from 5% to 9% in the United States, with an estimated 12-month prevalence of 2%.[15,16] The disability caused by GAD is thought to be approximately equal to that caused by major depressive disorder.[17] GAD is characterized by excessive worry or angst regarding several events or activities that one experiences daily. Symptoms must be present for at least 6 months and are experienced more days that not. These feelings are associated with at least 3 of the following additional symptoms: feelings of restlessness or being on edge, easy fatigability, trouble concentrating, irritability, muscle tension, and sleep disturbance. Diagnostic criteria maintain that symptoms are not explained by another psychiatric disorder or another medical condition. The worry affects daily functioning and produces disturbances in the daily routine of the patient.[18] Patients often present with somatic complaints, making diagnosis a challenge. More than 90% of patients suffering from GAD have a comorbid psychiatric diagnosis. A total of 48% of these patients are also suffering from major depressive disorder.[15] GAD is also frequently comorbid with medical disorders including chronic pain, headaches, irritable bowel syndrome, and sleep disorders.[5]

Characteristics associated with GAD include single marital status, female sex, multiple life stressors, lower educational level, and poor overall health.[19] Survey data suggest that even subthreshold symptoms of GAD can still significantly affect quality of life, causing considerable impairment of measures of human burden, which is defined as impairment in social, family, and occupational functioning; well-being; perceived emotional and physical health; and overall satisfaction with daily life.[20]

SOCIAL ANXIETY DISORDER

Social anxiety disorder (SAD), also known as social phobia, has an estimated lifetime morbidity risk of 13% and a 12-month prevalence of 7.4% in the United States.[16] The prominent feature of SAD is intense fear or anxiety of social situations in which the individual may risk being judged or scrutinized by others.[18] A specific SAD is the performance type, in which an individual experiences anxiety in his or her professional role, for example, performers or athletes, or in positions that require regular public speaking. Patients will experience physical symptoms such as trembling, sweating, blushing, or stuttering and are nervous about being criticized or rejected as a result. The degree of symptoms and how they handle the feared situations may vary between patients. Some individuals may rely on avoidance of the social setting, whereas others may suffer through the moment, all while enduring intense anxiety symptoms.[18]

The feelings an individual with SAD has are out of proportion to the real possibility of social scrutiny and may not be recognized by the individual. The care provider must be able to recognize this to make an accurate diagnosis. However, one must consider the cultural background of the patient, as what may appear to be increased social anxiety, for example, avoiding direct eye contact, may actually be a sign of respect in the patient's culture.[18]

PANIC DISORDER

Panic disorder has an estimated lifetime morbidity risk of 6.8% and a 12-month prevalence of 2.4%.[16] Symptoms are described as episodic panic attacks that are not necessarily elicited by one particular trigger.[21] Patients will suffer from sudden swells of acute and profound fear or discomfort accompanied by 4 or more of the following: palpitations, shortness of breath, sweating, chest pain, feelings of choking, trembling, nausea, dizziness, chills, paresthesias, depersonalization, or fear of dying or losing control.[18] Physical symptoms are paralyzing, leading to an abrupt disruption in the activity in which the individual was engaging. Patients with panic disorder will worry about having panic attacks, that is, where they will be when symptoms come on, who will be around to help them, and what others might think if they witness them having an attack. These pervasive thoughts may lead to maladaptive behavioral changes in which individuals avoid certain activities or locations for fear of having a panic attack. Agoraphobia may be present, in which case it should be made as a separate diagnosis.[18]

OBSESSIVE-COMPULSIVE DISORDER

Obsessive-compulsive disorder (OCD) now falls under the categorical heading of Obsessive-Compulsive and Related Disorders in the *Diagnostic and Statistical Manual of Mental Disorder, fifth edition*. Although logistically no longer classified as an anxiety disorder, the prevalence of OCD is high enough that primary care providers must be able to recognize and initiate treatment. The lifetime morbidity risk is 2.7% and the estimated 12-month prevalence is approximately 1.2%.[16] This disorder is marked by persistent and intrusive thoughts, such as, obsessions, and repetitive behaviors the patient feels compelled to perform, such as, compulsions.[22] The average time to diagnosis from symptom onset is approximately 11 years, which is partly because of the shame patients feel regarding their symptoms.[22] Symptoms can be of early or late onset, usually developing gradually, and are experienced as a continuous course.[22] One study found that patients who had early-onset symptoms suffered from higher lifetime rates of eating disorders, panic disorder, and obsessive-compulsive personality disorder.[22] The Yale-Brown Obsessive Compulsive Scale, a 10-item rater-administered measure of OCD symptoms, is the widely accepted major outcome measure for OCD.[22]

POSTTRAUMATIC STRESS DISORDER

PTSD can now be found in the category of Trauma and Stressor–Related Disorders of the *Diagnostic and Statistical Manual of Mental Disorder, fifth edition*, along with Acute Stress Disorder, Adjustment Disorders, Reactive Attachment Disorder, and Disinhibited Social Engagement Disorder. The estimated prevalence of PTSD in primary care is approximately 11.8%.[23] This disorder is marked by symptoms that develop after exposure to one or more traumatic events. These symptoms usually evolve within the first 3 months of the traumatic event but can be delayed for a period of months to years before they surface.[18] Clinical features of the disorder are described by 8 categories. The first highlights the inciting event—either direct exposure to the event, witnessing it happening to others, learning the event occurred to a close family member or friend, or being directly involved in the aftermath of the event (ie, first responders searching for survivors after the 9-11 attacks). Symptoms are invasive, recurrent, and focused around memories of the event. Dreams or flashbacks are common as is distress from a cue resembling the traumatic event. Patients will do their best to avoid stimuli that may trigger symptoms, and they often develop negative generalizations and assign them to other aspects of their lives, such as, "no one can be trusted." These negative feelings become a feature of their emotional state, as they carry anger, shame, or guilt and feel detached from others. Patients suffer from changes in arousal and reactivity and will often exhibit relatively unprovoked anger outbursts, hypervigilant states, concentration difficulty, and self-destructive behavior. The disturbance must be present for at least 1 month. The remaining criteria parallel those of other mental health disorders in that symptoms result in significant impairment in the patient's quality of life and are not caused by another medical condition or a substance.[18]

Rates of PTSD are typically highest for patients who have experienced military combat or captivity, rape, and "ethnically or politically motivated interment or genocide."[18] One study surveyed patients in a primary care setting and found the 3 "most upsetting" traumatic events were a life-threatening accident, being a witness to severe injury or death of others, and being a victim of sexual molestation.[23] PTSD is a chronic condition, and approximately one-third of patients may still experience symptoms up to 10 years after the inciting event.[24]

COMORBIDITY

Patients who experience 1 anxiety disorder commonly suffer from another psychiatric diagnosis, often another anxiety disorder.[1,4] Of note, patients suffering with more than one psychiatric diagnosis experience lower remission rates and increased rates of suicide.[5] The presence of more than one psychiatric disorder can make it challenging to treat anxiety. Although selective serotonin reuptake inhibitors (SSRIs) and serotonin-norepinephrine reuptake inhibitors (SNRIs) are approved as first-line treatment for both depression and anxiety, the delayed onset and variety of side effects can pose problems for patients with anxiety disorders.[5] For instance, a well-documented side effect of SSRIs is increased agitation and restlessness in the acute phase of treatment, often worsening anxiety symptoms.[15]

TREATMENT STRATEGIES
Selective Serotonin Reuptake Inhibitors and Serotonin-Norepinephrine Reuptake Inhibitors

Antidepressants are found to be effective in the treatment of anxiety disorders. The Cochrane Collaboration published a review in 2015 that examined the evidence for use of antidepressants for GAD. The study found that the use of imipramine, venlafaxine, and paroxetine are all superior to placebo in treating GAD, with a calculated number needed to treat (NNT) of 5.54.[25] SSRIs and SNRIs are by far considered the first-line agents in the treatment of anxiety. To date, no single SSRI or SNRI has been shown to be consistently more effective than another[15]; however, not all SSRIs carry the same US Food and Drug Administration (FDA) indications.[26] Of the 6 SSRIs (citalopram, escitalopram, fluoxetine, fluvoxamine, paroxetine, and sertraline), only sertraline and paroxetine are FDA approved for the treatment of SAD and PTSD.[26] Fluoxetine, in addition to paroxetine and sertraline, are the 3 SSRIs that are FDA approved for panic disorder.[26] Despite the varying FDA indications, all 6 SSRIs are often thought of by providers as having equal efficacy and are used as such in clinical practice.[26]

Although SSRIs are considered first-line treatment of anxiety disorders for their efficacy and tolerability, they still carry significant side effects. At the time of initiation of SSRIs, patients may experience headaches, nausea, jitteriness, and dizziness, symptoms that are often mistaken for worsening anxiety symptoms and therefore interfere with adherence.[15,26] These medications should be started at low doses, titrated slowly to the higher end of the dose range, and continued for at least 4 weeks before the patient should expect significant symptom relief.[21] Once the medication has taken effect and symptoms are subsiding, it should be continued for at least 1 year before attempting to taper.[27]

SNRIs can also be used to treat anxiety disorders. Venlafaxine ER is the SNRI most studied in the treatment of anxiety and is currently approved for GAD, panic disorder, and SAD.[26] Duloxetine is also approved for GAD.[26] Both SSRIs and SNRIs may also provoke a discontinuation syndrome, and it is important to think about tapering these medications gradually or choosing one with a longer half-life.[26] Treatment of anxiety disorders may require higher doses of SSRIs or SNRIs and longer duration of treatment than indicated for depression.[28]

Tricyclic Antidepressants and Monoamine Oxidase Inhibitors

Tricyclic antidepressants (TCAs) are another option in the management of anxiety disorders[15]; however, the evidence supporting their efficacy varies.[26] TCAs have been studied in panic disorder, generalized anxiety disorder, PTSD, and OCD.

Clomipramine and imipramine have both been shown to be more effective than placebo for panic disorder.[26] Imipramine was compared with diazepam and was found to be an effective anxiolytic in the treatment of generalized anxiety disorder, although with more reported side effects than diazepam.[26] Currently, clomipramine is considered the gold standard treatment for OCD, however, only after an SSRI has been tried first.[26] The major disadvantage of TCAs is their side-effect profile, which includes antiadrenergic and anticholinergic symptoms such as dry mouth, constipation, sedation, sexual dysfunction, and orthostatic hypotension.[26] These symptoms are common, and often intolerable, and are the main reasons TCAs reside as a third- or fourth-line option in the treatment of anxiety.[26]

As with TCAs, monoamine oxidase inhibitors (MAOIs) exist as yet another option when treatment with SSRIs or SNRIs has failed. However, the use of MAOIs has fallen out of favor because of their risk of hypertensive crises when tyramine is not avoided and their interference with other medications.[26] MAOIs should be initiated with caution in patients with resistant anxiety after treatment with mainstay options. Careful consideration should be given to referring these patients to a psychiatrist.

Buspirone

Buspirone shows anxiolytic effects by acting as a partial agonist to the 5-HT$_{1A}$ receptor.[26] Buspirone is the only agent in the azapirone class that is approved for the treatment of anxiety, particularly GAD.[26] It seems to be particularly useful in patients with chronic anxiety that does not respond to benzodiazepines.[29] It is generally well tolerated and has a low potential for dependence. However, buspirone takes approximately 2 to 3 weeks to take effect.[30]

Benzodiazepines

Benzodiazepines (BZDs) are successful agents in mitigating acute anxiety symptoms and are rapidly acting, effective, and well tolerated.[15] Benzodiazepines are often used in the acute anxiety phase as a means to bridging to more long-term agents, such as SSRIs or SNRIs, and can also be used during periods of symptom exacerbation.[15] BZDs act on the γ-amino-butyric acid/benzodiazepine receptor complex resulting in muscle relaxation, sedation, and decreased awareness.[11] Agents with longer half-lives, such as clonazepam (50 hours), are often preferred, as the doses are less frequent and they are advantageous at limiting anxiety symptoms between doses. Shorter-acting options may be preferred in geriatric patients, as they tend to cause less sedation and are more easily metabolized.[11] These agents include oxazepam, alprazolam, and lorazepam, with half-lives of 14 hours, 14 hours, and 9 hours, respectively.[11] The shorter half-lives offer the benefit of dosing on an as-needed basis, for example, before a flight or in a patient with specific phobia.

Despite the effectiveness of BZDs in acute anxiety, clinicians should be wary of prescribing these agents long term. Risk for dependence and abuse is high, especially for agents that are more rapidly absorbed, and withdrawal and rebound symptoms are common if abruptly discontinued.[15] Although BZDs are more desirable in the acute phase, antidepressants are found to reach and even surpass the efficacy of BZDs at 6 to 12 weeks of treatment and therefore continue to be preferred as first-line treatment.[31,32]

Other Second-Line Agents

In addition to the above first-line agents for treatment of anxiety disorders, **Table 2** outlines second- and third-line agents including hydroxyzine for panic disorder or

GAD, antipsychotics or antiepileptics for GAD, and β-blockers for SAD. A myriad of agents available for augmentation are also noted.

Second-generation antipsychotics, in particular, have been used extensively in the treatment of anxiety disorders. Although little robust data exist for most of the second-generation antipsychotics, quetiapine does seem to be effective as monotherapy for GAD. Unfortunately, the most common side effects—weight gain and sedation—often limit its use. Nonetheless, quetiapine remains an option for uncomplicated GAD.

Special Populations

Table 3 summarizes pharmacology treatment considerations for particular patient groups.

Nonpharmacologic Strategies

There are several nonpharmacologic treatment options available for patients with anxiety disorders. Cognitive behavioral therapy (CBT) is perhaps the most validated non-pharmacologic approach for anxiety disorders, although the particular technique may differ for each diagnosis. For example, exposure therapy predominates as the theme in SAD. The idea is that with repeated exposure to the social situation, symptoms will diminish with time, and patients will be able to tolerate what they could not before.[33]

Common CBT strategies for GAD include self-monitoring of anxiety, in which patients are instructed to imagine anxiety-provoking situations and notice what they are feeling, both physically and mentally. The goal is for the patient to be able to recognize these cues early and implement coping mechanisms before being overcome by anxiety symptoms.[34] Relaxation training, cognitive therapy, and imagery rehearsal of coping skills are other techniques useful in GAD.[34]

Exposure and response prevention is found to be effective in the treatment of OCD.[35] Individuals are exposed to situations that provoke fear related to their obsessions and are taught to suppress their usual compulsive actions (ie, exposure to a cluttered, disorganized desk and controlling the need or desire to organize it).[35] Patients with severe symptoms may require CBT administered by a mental health professional over a longer period of time, usually 13 to 20 sessions each lasting about 1 to 2 hours.[36]

CBT for panic disorder takes a similar approach to that for other anxiety disorders. The goal is that, over time, the patient is able to recognize his thought process as inaccurate and exaggerated and restructure these patterns of thinking into more realistic realizations of the situation and then adapt accordingly.[37] A recent randomized controlled trial compared CBT with panic-focused psychodynamic psychotherapy and applied relaxation training in the treatment of panic disorder and found that all treatments were effective, with CBT proving to be the most consistently effective option.[38]

Although CBT is found to be as effective, if not more so, than medication in the treatment of some anxiety disorders, currently evidence is insufficient to suggest psychotherapy is more effective in treating PTSD than pharmacotherapy.[39] Examples of some specific therapies used in PTSD include prolonged exposure, cognitive processing, and eye movement desensitization and reprocessing. These therapies are composed of elements such as narrative exposure, in vivo exposure by directly confronting the trigger, cognitive restructuring, and relaxation techniques.[39,40] Hypnosis, imagery rehearsal, and brief psychodynamic therapy are other alternative therapies.[40]

Psychotherapy administered in a primary care setting is usually more brief than that provided by a mental health specialist because of time constraints. For example, a

Table 2
Treatment options

Anxiety Disorder	First-Line Agents	Second-Line Agents	Third-Line Agents	Augmentation	Nonpharmacologic Options	Additional Considerations
Panic disorder	SSRIs • Escitalopram • Fluoxetine • Fluvoxamine • Paroxetine • Sertraline SNRIs • Venlafaxine • Duloxetine	TCAs • Amitriptyline • Imipramine • Nortriptyline Hydroxyzine	MAOIs • Isocarboxazid • Phenelzine • Tranylcypromine	Benzodiazepines • Alprazolam • Clonazepam • Lorazepam	CBT Exercise	CBT + medication yields the best outcomes
GAD	SSRIs • Escitalopram • Fluoxetine • Paroxetine • Sertraline SNRIs • Venlafaxine • Duloxetine Azapirone • Buspirone	TCAs • Amitriptyline • Imipramine • Nortriptyline Antiepileptics • Pregabalin Antipsychotics • Quetiapine Hydroxyzine	MAOIs • Isocarboxazid • Phenelzine • Tranylcypromine	Benzodiazepines • Alprazolam • Clonazepam • Lorazepam • Diazepam	CBT focusing on the role of worrying and avoidance behavior	BZDs should be used with caution after other treatments have failed
SAD	SSRIs • Fluoxetine • Paroxetine • Sertraline • Fluvoxamine • Citalopram SNRIs Venlafaxine	Beta-blockers • Propranolol • Nadolol • Atenolol	MAOIs • Phenelzine • Tranylcypromine	Benzodiazepines • Alprazolam • Lorazepam • Clonazepam	CBT Exposure therapy	Although sometimes used for augmentation, BZDs have not been extensively studied No evidence for TCAs Phenelzine (irreversible MAOI) can be used in resistant cases

OCD	SSRIs • Citalopram • Escitalopram • Fluoxetine • Fluvoxamine • Paroxetine • Sertraline TCAs • Clomipramine SNRIs • Venlafaxine	—	CBT Exposure and response prevention	Requires long-term treatment Deep brain stimulation is an option
PTSD	SSRIs • Citalopram • Escitalopram • Fluoxetine • Paroxetine • Sertraline SNRIs • Venlafaxine • Desvenlafaxine • Duloxetine TCAs • Amitriptyline • Clomipramine • Desipramine • Imipramine • Nortriptyline Doxepin Mirtazapine Trazodone	MAOIs • Phenelzine Antiadrenergic • Clonidine • Guanfacine • Prazosin • Propranolol Mood stabilizers/anticonvulsants • Carbamazepine • Gabapentin • Lamotrigine • Lithium • Topiramate • Valproate Other agents • Buspirone • Diphenhydramine • Zaleplon • Zolpidem	CBT Trauma-focused therapies including narrative exposure and in vivo exposure	Requires long-term treatment (12–24 mo) Long-term efficacy proven for fluoxetine, sertraline and venlafaxine "Debriefing" and BZDs are contraindicated in the first few hours after exposure, as they may interfere with the natural recovery process

Data from Refs.[21,34,39,49]

Table 3 Special treatment considerations	
Pregnancy	• No apparent increased risk of malformations with SSRIs and TCAs • Avoid paroxetine and alprazolam in pregnant women or those planning to become pregnant.
Breast feeding	• SSRIs and TCAs are excreted into breast milk and have been detected in infants' serum. • No current recommendation to discontinue breast feeding if being treated with SSRIs or TCAs. • If breast feeding mother is treated with BZDs, need to monitor infant for sedation, poor suckling, weight loss, and lethargy; may need to discontinue breast feeding if higher doses of BZDs are required.
Treatment of children and adolescents	• SSRIs are first line. • Should be evaluated for comorbid depression owing to warnings regarding increased risk of suicidal ideation.
Treatment of the elderly	• SSRIs are safest. • TCAs and BZDs should be used with caution because of increased risk of side effects including anticholinergic effects, orthostatic hypotension, electrocardiogram changes with TCAs, and possibility for depression, aggressiveness, or violent behavior and phobias with BZD treatment.
Treatment of patients with severe somatic disease	• Avoid TCAs in patients with cardiac disease. • SSRIs are better in patients with cardiac disease. • Monitor blood pressure closely in patients with underlying hypertension taking venlafaxine.

From Bandelow B, Sher L, Bunevicius R, et al. Guidelines for the pharmacological treatment of anxiety disorders, obsessive-compulsive disorder and posttraumatic stress disorder in primary care. Int J Psychiatry Clin Pract 2012;16:77–84; with permission.

usual duration of psychotherapy treatment in the United Kingdom in a primary care setting is roughly 6 sessions, as compared to well-studied and efficacious 12 to 24 sessions.[41] A meta-analysis found that brief CBT for anxiety disorders was comparable to the effectiveness of longer treatments in primary care.[41] The analysis also found that brief counseling and problem-solving therapy were also effective although not as effective as those treatments given over a longer period of time.[41] A randomized controlled trial conducted in the Netherlands found that patients with prevalent anxiety disorders, particularly panic disorder and generalized anxiety disorder, could be adequately treated by their general practitioner in a primary care setting, and referral to a psychiatrist did not yield better results.[42]

Other nonpharmacologic therapies documented to have some success in the treatment of anxiety include mindfulness-based meditation, muscle relaxation, and breathing exercises.[4] Yoga and exercise are also found to be superior to no treatment.[43] These options are more effective if used as adjunctive therapies to the mainstays of treatment.

Alternative Medicine

Many other treatments for anxiety disorder have been described in the literature. Kava extract is found to be an effective remedy, although case reports of hepatotoxicity have discouraged its use.[6] St. John's wort is another agent reported to treat anxiety; however, it has significant drug interaction potential, as it is metabolized through the cytochrome P450 system. In particular, it may trigger serotonin syndrome through interactions with other serotonergic agents.[4]

Collaborative Care

Ideally, offering treatment for anxiety in primary care should occur in the context of a functioning collaborative care model. This model centers around a care manager, often a social worker or a registered nurse, who is responsible for keeping in close contact with the patient while working as a liaison between the primary care physician and the patient's mental health provider. The care manager may perform various monitoring functions, both therapeutic and psychoeducational, to help facilitate a more comprehensive, holistic treatment plan.[44]

Although most research on collaborative care thus far has focused on depression,[44] evidence suggests it is a successful technique in the treatment of anxiety disorders as well. Katon and colleagues[45] found that a collaborative care intervention was associated with significantly more anxiety-free days in patients with panic disorder. A recent randomized controlled trial examined this approach in 4 anxiety disorders: GAD, panic disorder, PTSD, and SAD.[46] This study found that the CALM (Coordinated Anxiety Learning and Management) model led to a statistically significant improvement in symptoms in patients with anxiety disorders compared with usual care from primary care providers.[46] A follow-up qualitative study investigated barriers to and facilitators of this approach, that is, why was the CALM model so successful and what obstacles would prevent its implementation in all clinics?[44] The most common implementation barrier was difficulty with physician buy-in or motivation to participate. This barrier was hypothesized to be caused by to variation in physician interest in mental health issues and underestimation of the prevalence of mental health disorders within his or her clinic. Other barriers included the physical structure of the clinic, such as, space constraints for anxiety clinical specialists and reimbursement issues related the model. Facilitators to implementation were many, including the idea that most patients preferred a "one-stop shop" — they liked being able to come to their PCPs office for mental health services. Provider enthusiasm increased when somatic complaints of patients were noticeably reduced. The CALM model also seemed to work well if the care center already had a mental health provider in house or if collaborative care services were already established in the clinic for another mental health disorder. The model was more successful when anxiety clinical specialists worked full time and were easily accessible to the rest of the care team.[44] The next step in this research is to study this model under more practical circumstances, such as, when it is not paid for by research funding.[44]

Military primary care has been the site for the development of collaborative care models to address both depression and PTSD. The RESPECT-Mil project (Re-Engineering Systems of Primary Care Treatment in the Military) is a collaborative care model that was implemented within US Army primary care clinics. Notable findings include a 93% screening rate (depression and PTSD) of service members, a 13% positive screen rate, and a 61% probable mental health diagnosis rate. In addition, impressive treatment response rates were found (42% of depressed soldiers showed at least a 50% symptom reduction through last follow-up; 33% of soldiers with PTSD showed at least a 50% symptom reduction through last follow-up).[47] The STEPS-UP trial (Stepped Enhancement of PTSD Services Using Primary Care) is the first large randomized effectiveness trial to be completed in US military primary care clinics. Although initial effectiveness results have not been released, the findings of this study promise to better inform the nature of effective primary care collaborative care approaches within military (and civilian) settings.[48]

Discussion

Given the high prevalence of anxiety disorders in the general population, primary care providers should be well equipped to recognize the diagnosis and initiate management. Although screening may not be recommended for all patients, it is certainly warranted in patients presenting with concerning symptoms, or those with multiple somatic complaints whose workup has been unsuccessful in defining a clear medical etiology. Despite the differences in diagnostic criteria for each anxiety disorder, treatment is generally the same. Before starting treatment, it is important to recognize that many patients suffering with anxiety may have a comorbid mental health disorder. SSRIs and SNRIs remain first-line agents for the chronic management of these mental health disorders. Other options include TCAs, MAOIs, and buspirone. Augmenting with antipsychotics is an option in resistant cases. However, once patients have progressed to needing these medications, it may be best to collaborate with a psychiatrist for further management assistance. Benzodiazepines are highly effective at treating acute anxiety symptoms and can be used to help bridge patients in the initial period after starting SSRIs, as they may experience worsening anxiety during this time. Psychotherapy is found to be effective as a treatment option alone or in conjunction with medication. Ideally, treatment of anxiety and other mental health disorders should be carried out in a setting in which the appropriate systems are in place to treat patients on a long-term basis. The collaborative care model is found to be effective in this way for major depressive disorder, and recent studies show its effectiveness for anxiety as well.

REFERENCES

1. Kroenke K, Spitzer FL, Williams JBW, et al. Anxiety disorders in primary care: prevalence, impairment, comorbidity, and detection. Ann Intern Med 2007;146: 317–25.
2. Kessler RC, Berglund P, Demler O, et al. Lifetime prevalence and age-of-onset distributions of DSM-IV disorders in the National Comorbidity Survey Replication. Arch Gen Psychiatry 2005;62(6):593–602.
3. Saarni SI, Suvisaari J, Sintonen H, et al. Impact of psychiatric disorders on health-related quality of life: general population survey. Br J Psychiatry 2007;190: 326–32.
4. Combs H, Markman J. Anxiety disorders in primary care. Med Clin North Am 2014;98:1007–23.
5. Nutt D, Argyropoulos S, Hood S, et al. Generalized anxiety disorder: a comorbid disease. Eur Neuropsychopharmacol 2006;16(Suppl 2):S109–18.
6. Narayana S, Wong CJ. Office-based screening of common psychiatric conditions. Med Clin North Am 2014;98:959–80.
7. Broadhead WE, Leon AC, Weissman MM, et al. Development and validation of the SDDS-PC screen for multiple mental disorders in primary care. Arch Fam Med 1995;4:211–9.
8. Prins A, Ouimette P, Kimerling R, et al. The primary care PTSD screen (PC-PTSD): development and operating characteristics. Prim Care Psychiatr 2003; 9:9–14.
9. Freedy JR, Steenkamp MM, Magruder KM, et al. Post-traumatic stress disorder screening test performance in civilian primary care. Fam Pract 2010;27: 615–24.

10. Simon GE, Von Korff M, Piccinelli M, et al. An international study of the relation between somatic symptoms and depression. N Engl J Med 1999;341:1329–35.
11. Gliatto MF. Generalized anxiety disorder. Am Fam Physician 2000;62(7): 1591–600.
12. Kroenke K. Patients presenting with somatic complaints: epidemiology, psychiatric co-morbidity and management. Int J Methods Psychiatr Res 2003;12(1): 34–43.
13. Kroenke K, Spitzer RL, Williams JBW, et al. Physical symptoms in primary care: predictors of psychiatric disorders and functional impairment. Arch Fam Med 1994;3:774–9.
14. Wise MG, Griffies WS. A combined treatment approach to anxiety in the medically ill. J Clin Psychiatry 1995;56(suppl 2):14–9.
15. Reinhold JA, Mados LA, Rickels K, et al. Pharmacological treatment of generalized anxiety disorder. Expert Opin Pharmacother 2011;12(16):2457–67.
16. Kessler RC, Petukhova M, Sampson NA, et al. Twelve-month and lifetime prevalence and lifetime morbid risk of anxiety and mood disorders in the United States. Int J Methods Psychiatr Res 2012;21(3):169–84.
17. Kessler RC, DuPont RL, Berglund P, et al. Impairment in pure and comorbid generalized anxiety disorder and major depression at 12 months in two national surveys. Am J Psychiatry 1999;156(12):1915–23.
18. American Psychiatric Association. Diagnostic and statistical manual of mental disorders. 5th edition. Washington, DC: American Psychiatric Association; 2013.
19. Wolitzky-Taylor KB, Castriotta N, Lenze EJ, et al. Anxiety disorders in older adults: a comprehensive review. Depress Anxiety 2010;27(2):190–211.
20. Kertz SJ, Woodruff-Borden J. Human and economic burden of GAD, subthreshold GAD, and worry in a primary care group practice. J Clin Psychol Med Settings 2011;18(3):281–90.
21. Locke AB, Kirst N, Shultz CG. Diagnosis and management of generalized anxiety disorder and panic disorder in adults. Am Fam Physician 2015;91(9):617–24.
22. Pinto A, Mancebo MC, Eisen JL, et al. The brown longitudinal obsessive compulsive study: clinical features and symptoms of the sample at intake. J Clin Psychiatry 2006;67(5):703–11.
23. Stein MB, McQuaid JR, Pedrelli P, et al. Posttraumatic stress disorder in the primary care medical setting. Gen Hosp Psychiatry 2000;22(4):261–9.
24. Kessler RC, Sonnega A, Bromet E, et al. Posttraumatic stress disorder in the National Comorbidity Survey. Arch Gen Psychiatry 1995;52(12):1048–60.
25. Kapczinski F, Lima MS, Souza JS, et al. Antidepressants for generalized anxiety disorder. Cochrane Database Syst Rev 2003;(2):CD003592.
26. Ravindran LN, Stein MB. The pharmacologic treatment of anxiety disorders: a review of progress. J Clin Psychiatry 2010;71(7):839–54.
27. National Institute for Health and Care Excellence. Generalised anxiety disorder and panic disorder (with or without agoraphobia) in adults: management in primary, secondary and community care. Available at: http://www.nice.org.uk/Guidance/CG113. Accessed January 4, 2016.
28. Stahl S. Stahl's essential psychopharmacology: the prescriber's guide. New York: Cambridge University Press; 2011.
29. Rickels K, Schweizer E. The clinical course and long-term management of generalized anxiety disorder. J Clin Psychopharmacol 1990;10:101S–10S.

30. Longo LP. Non-benzodiazepine pharmacotherapy of anxiety and panic in substance abusing patients. Psychiatr Ann 1998;28:142–53.

31. Rickels K, Downing R, Schweizer E, et al. Antidepressants for the treatment of generalized anxiety disorder. A placebo-controlled comparison of imipramine, trazodone and diazepam. Arch Gen Psychiatry 1993;50:884–95.

32. Rickels K, Zaninelli R, McCafferty J, et al. Paroxetine treatment of generalized anxiety disorder: a double-blind, placebo-controlled study. Am J Psychiatry 2003;10:749–56.

33. Barlow D, Barlow D. Clinical handbook of psychological disorders. New York: Guilford Press; 2008.

34. Bruce TJ, Saeed SA. Social anxiety disorder: a common, underrecognized mental disorder. Am Fam Physician 1999;60(8):2311–20.

35. Koran LM, Hanna GL, Hollander E, et al, American Psychiatric Association. Practice guideline for the treatment of patients with obsessive-compulsive disorder. Am J Psychiatry 2007;164(7 Suppl):5–53.

36. Fisher PL, Wells A. How effective are cognitive and behavioral treatments for obsessive-compulsive disorder? A clinical significant analysis. Behav Res Ther 2005;43(12):1543–58.

37. Smits JAJ, Powers MB, Cho Y, et al. Mechanism of change in cognitive-behavioral treatment of panic disorder: evidence for the fear of fear mediational hypothesis. J Consult Clin Psychol 2004;72(4):646–52.

38. Milrod B, Chambless DL, Gallop R, et al. Psychotherapies for panic disorder: a tale of two sites. J Clin Psychiatry 2015. [Epub ahead of print].

39. Warner CH, Warner CM, Appenzeller GN, et al. Identifying and managing post-traumatic stress disorder. Am Fam Physician 2013;88(12):827–34.

40. Department of Veterans Affairs; Department of Defense. VA/DoD clinical practice guideline for the management of post-traumatic stress. Available at: http://www.healthquality.va.gov/ptsd/cpg_PTSD-FULL-201011612.pdf. Accessed August 1, 2015.

41. Cape J, Whittington C, Buszewicz M, et al. Brief psychological therapies for anxiety and depression in primary care: meta-analysis and meta-regression. BMC Med 2010;8:38.

42. van Boeijen CA, van Oppen P, van Balkom AJ, et al. Treatment of anxiety disorders in primary care practice: a randomized controlled trial. Br J Gen Pract 2005;55:763–9.

43. Saeed SY, Antonacci DJ, Bloch RM. Exercise, yoga, and meditation for depressive and anxiety disorders. Am Fam Physician 2010;81(8):981–6.

44. Curran GM, Sullivan G, Mendel P, et al. Implementation of the CALM intervention for anxiety disorders: a qualitative study. Implement Sci 2012;7:14.

45. Katon WJ, Roy-Byrne P, Russo J, et al. Cost-effectiveness and cost offset of a collaborative care intervention for primary care patients with panic disorder. Arch Gen Psychiatry 2002;59(12):1098–104.

46. Roy-Byrne PP, Craske MG, Sullivan G, et al. Delivery of evidence-based treatment for multiple anxiety disorders in primary care: a randomized controlled trial. JAMA 2010;303:1921–8.

47. Wong EC, Jaycox LH, Ayer L, et al. Evaluating the Implementation of the Re-Engineering Systems of Primary Care Treatment in the Military (RESPECT-Mil). Santa Monica (CA): Rand Corporation; 2015.

48. Engel CC, Bray RM, Jaycox LH, et al. Implementing collaborative primary care for depression and posttraumatic stress disorder: design and sample for a randomized trial in the U.S. military health system. Contemp Clin Trials 2014;39(2): 310–9.
49. Bandelow B, Sher L, Bunevicius R, et al. Guidelines for the pharmacological treatment of anxiety disorders, obsessive-compulsive disorder and posttraumatic stress disorder in primary care. Int J Psychiatry Clin Pract 2012;16:77–84.

Pearls for Working with People Who Have Personality Disorder Diagnoses

 CrossMark

Gene Combs, MD[a],*, Lauren Oshman, MD, MPH[b]

KEYWORDS

- Personality disorder • Borderline personality disorder • Cluster B
- Motivational interviewing • Dialectical behavior therapy

KEY POINTS

- There is lack of general agreement and empirical evidence on how best to categorize personality problems.
- Primary care physicians should exercise great caution before assigning a personality disorder diagnosis; they should look closely at their relationship with the person in question and not use a diagnostic label to blame a patient for what is better conceptualized as a relationship problem.
- The bulk of the literature on working with personality disorders in primary care focuses on borderline personality disorder, a cluster B category.
- Primary care physicians can use principles and practices from motivational interviewing and dialectical behavior therapy to relate to people who show borderline personality disorder or cluster B traits.

INTRODUCTION

People with personality disorder diagnoses use primary care services at a higher rate than the general population.[1] People with personality disorder diagnoses are at increased risk for suicide, substance abuse, accidental injury, depression, and homicide.[2] Although there seems to be general agreement that people have personalities, and that personalities can be disordered, there is considerable controversy over how to best name and describe personality disorders. The *Diagnostic and Statistical Manual of Mental Disorders* (DSM) of the American Psychiatric Association asks clinicians to sort people who show personality characteristics that significantly and adversely affect

[a] Departments of Family Medicine and Psychiatry, NorthShore University HealthSystem, Glenbrook Hospital, University of Chicago, Suite 200, 2050 Pfingsten Road, Glenview, IL 60025, USA; [b] Department of Family Medicine, NorthShore University HealthSystem, Glenbrook Hospital, University of Chicago, Suite 200, 2050 Pfingsten Road, Glenview, IL 60025, USA
* Corresponding author. Department of Family Medicine, NorthShore University HealthSystem, Glenbrook Hospital, University of Chicago, Suite 200, 2050 Pfingsten Road, Glenview, IL 60025.
E-mail address: gcombs@northshore.org

Prim Care Clin Office Pract 43 (2016) 263–268
http://dx.doi.org/10.1016/j.pop.2016.02.001   **primarycare.theclinics.com**
0095-4543/16/$ – see front matter © 2016 Elsevier Inc. All rights reserved.

many aspects of their lives into specific "personality disorder" categories. It lists specific criteria that must be satisfied before a person can be assigned to a personality disorder category. The mere existence of these categories, and their sanctioning by the American Psychiatric Association,[3] can lead clinicians all too easily to forget that personality disorders are not diseases in any classical sense, and that there is considerable lack of agreement about the best way to describe and assess them. A 2007 review article states, "The assessment of personality disorder is currently inaccurate, largely unreliable, frequently wrong and in need of improvement."[4] As DSM-5 went to press, there was still substantial disagreement about how to categorize personality disorders—so much so that an alternative classification system was included in an appendix.[5] Because of these uncertainties, this article focuses more on broad principles than on detailed descriptions of the diagnosis and treatment of each and every DSM or International Classification of Diseases category of personality disorder.

It is important to remember that every clinical relationship has at least two participants, and that when things become interpersonally difficult, all of the involved parties bear some responsibility for the difficulty. When it seems that the clinician might be dealing with a disordered personality, he or she must reflect on his or her own contribution to what is happening moment-by-moment in that particular clinical encounter. Although the literature on working with personality disorders tends to focus on "difficult patients," it is more accurate and useful to think in terms of "difficult doctor-patient relationships."[6,7] Before deciding that any person who comes to a clinician for help should be diagnosed with a personality disorder, one needs to take a careful look at his or her relationship with that person, and at how the clinician might be bringing forth certain aspects of the patient's personality and not leaving room for others. One must understand enough about the total context of a person's life to know that the traits they show within the clinical relationship occur to a significant degree in other relationships, and that they have done so for a long time.

SCREENING AND DIAGNOSIS

Routine screening for personality disorders is not recommended, and a personality disorder should only be formally and officially diagnosed when clear, pervasive, and persistent difficulties result from aspects of a person's personality. Even then, because they can be stigmatizing, care should be exercised as to how these labels are mentioned in medical records and in communication with others.

Although the most widely used system for classifying personality disorders is the DSM-5, there is much contention as to the usefulness or accuracy of this system. In the DSM-5, the general requirements for a diagnosis of personality disorder are as follows:

- Significant impairments in functioning as it relates to personality.
- The impairments are relatively stable across time and consistent across situations.
- The impairments are not better understood as normative for the individual's developmental stage or sociocultural environment.
- The impairments are not solely caused by the direct physiologic effects of a substance or a general medical condition.

The criteria for specific personality disorders must meet all of these criteria, as well as Cluster A, B, and C personality disorder criteria outlined in the DSM-5.[3]

The 10 personality disorders are grouped into three clusters: cluster A (paranoid, schizoid, and schizotypal), cluster B (antisocial, borderline, histrionic, and narcissistic), and cluster C (avoidant, dependent, and obsessive-compulsive). Because there is considerable overlap among the subtypes in each cluster, there is greater interrater reliability for assignment to clusters than for assignment to specific disorder type. Most of the evidence concerning effective treatment comes from studies based on the three clusters.[5] Most difficulties in day-to-day clinical practice occur with people who are seen as exhibiting cluster B traits, and the most problematic of these people will likely be assigned a label of borderline personality disorder at some point in their clinical history.

MANAGEMENT GOALS

In primary care, the goal is rarely to treat a personality disorder itself; rather, the goal is much more often to manage some other disease process or health concern. Providers become concerned about a personality disorder when behaviors and attitudes, such as distrust, irritability, dependency, and excessive-seeming demands, get in the way of other clinical goals.[8] Hardly any high-level evidence exists concerning the treatment of personality disorders or the management of people with personality disorder diagnoses in clinical practice. The recommendations in this article, except where more specific citations are given, are drawn from reviews of expert opinion.[9–12]

The first-line treatment of personality disorders is psychotherapy, and there is good support in the literature for the efficacy of several forms of psychotherapy in regard to borderline personality disorder.[5] Primary care physicians usually do not take on the role of psychotherapist; but referral to a psychotherapist, and active consultation that includes that therapist as an ongoing member of the overall health care team, is an important part of successful management. The principles in **Box 1** help in negotiating acceptance of referral to a therapist.

Box 1
Expert guidelines for people with cluster B traits

Because of their difficulties in controlling emotions, their exquisite sensitivity to anything that feels like abandonment, and their tendency toward all-or-nothing thinking, it is hard for people with borderline personality disorder traits to engage in and stick with a treatment plan. The following principles can help:

- Use a team approach. Actively consult with at least one other person when things get difficult.
- Maintain clear, unambiguous communication with the patient and with all persons on the treatment team.
- Explore treatment options in an atmosphere of hope and optimism.
- Work in an open, engaging, and nonjudgmental manner to build a trusting relationship.
- Remember that people with cluster B diagnoses usually come from a life history of trauma, rejection, abuse, and neglect, so that they are especially sensitive to slights and stigmatization.
- Expect emotional volatility and cultivate calmness in the face of it.
- Do not become overly impressed by intense or dramatic praise nor overly discouraged by harsh criticism.
- Support the person in finding solutions for life problems, but calmly, compassionately give them primary responsibility for problem resolution.
- Encourage the person to identify manageable short-term goals and to specify steps to take in reaching them.

The chief management goal in every situation involving personality disorder diagnoses is that of maintaining a useful and fulfilling doctor-patient relationship. Personality disorder diagnoses should not be used as a subtle, professional-sounding form of name calling, or as a way of blaming patients for clinicians' difficulties in responding to them. Most clinicians do reasonably well at maintaining their emotional balance with people who would fit in cluster A or cluster C. However, people with cluster B traits present more of a challenge, especially in the case of borderline personality disorder. Some generalizations can be made according to cluster type about common problems and considerations in managing the doctor-patient relationship with people who present with strong personality disorder traits.

People who fulfill criteria for grouping under cluster A (paranoid, schizoid, and schizotypal) have seemed odd or eccentric to enough people in enough situations to warrant such grouping. This means that physicians need to allow for their idiosyncrasies and not be discouraged or put off by them. They offer an opportunity to work on skills of patience, persistence, and kindness. A professional stance, clear explanations, and extra effort to tolerate odd beliefs and behaviors are recommended.[7,13]

Cluster B (antisocial, borderline, histrionic, narcissistic) is the grouping for people who others experience as problematically dramatic, emotional, and/or erratic. To be effective partners for them, clinicians need to work as a coordinated team and support each other in staying calm and consistent in the face of dramatic and quickly changing emotions and life situations. Frequently mentioned expert guidelines for dealing with cluster B personalities are listed in **Box 1**. Some forms of psychotherapy have been found helpful for borderline personality disorder.[14] Dialectical behavior therapy has been most studied and has the strongest evidence supporting it. Other therapies with single-study support for effectiveness are mentalization-based therapy, transference-focused therapy, and interpersonal therapy.

People who qualify for a cluster C (avoidant, dependent, and obsessive-compulsive) designation have been seen as anxious or fearful in life-limiting ways. Such people need a calming, reliable, and reassuring approach from their clinician.

PHARMACOLOGIC STRATEGIES

Although drugs are sometimes used to lessen emotional and interpersonal distress in people with personality disorder diagnoses, no drug is specifically approved as a direct treatment of any personality disorder. All use of drugs in the treatment of people deserving of a personality disorder diagnosis is for symptoms, such as selective serotonin reuptake inhibitors or benzodiazepines aimed at anxiety; general central nervous system damping-down agents, such as antiepileptic drugs and antipsychotic drugs, aimed at overreactivity; and stimulant drugs aimed at low energy or difficulties with attention. People with personality disorders are more sensitive to side effects, tend to take more of a drug than prescribed, and are at increased risk for using street drugs and alcohol.[6] Drugs are not curative for any personality disorder. They should be viewed as an adjunct and used only for clear target symptoms, in the lowest effective doses, and discontinued as soon as possible.[12] Clinicians should carefully consider individual risks and benefits, including side effects, drug-drug interactions, and teratogenicity, when prescribing these medications.

SELF-MANAGEMENT STRATEGIES

Angstman and Rasmussen[12] have recommended a motivational interviewing–based approach for primary care physicians in helping people manage the problems of

Table 1
Step-by-step implementation of motivational interviewing

Step	Example
Ask for permission to discuss the problem.	Would it be okay for us to talk about scheduling your appointments?
Invite talk about change: Are things OK the way they are? What would make the situation better? Are there any realistic steps that could be taken to lessen the problem?	It seems like you have been frustrated when you call and can't get in to see me immediately, is that true? Do you think that scheduling our appointments closer together would make it less likely that you'll have to deal with that kind of frustration? Do you have any other ideas about how we might make it less frustrating?
Check the importance of changing.	On a scale of 1–10 how important is it to have predictable times for when we can meet?
Check the perceived ability to change.	On a scale of 1–10 how confident are you that you can keep once-a-week appointments if we make them? Do you think having weekly appointments will decrease the need for unscheduled urgent appointments?
Summarize: Review the problem, any commitments that have been made, and any questions or unresolved issues that remain.	So, let's review what we've said here. We have both had some frustration over scheduling. You haven't been able to see me a quickly as you wanted at times, and we have been dealing with little emergencies rather than working out a smooth overall plan for dealing with your problems. We're going to try scheduling weekly appointments to see if that helps us get on top of things so that there are fewer situations that feel really urgent to you. We're not sure if that will solve the whole problem, but we'll see what difference it makes. How does that fit with your understanding?

Adapted from Angstman KB, Rasmussen NH. Personality disorders: review and clinical application in daily practice. Am Fam Physician 2011;84(11):1253–60.

personality disorders. **Table 1** illustrates a step-by-step application of motivational interviewing principles in a person with cluster B traits.

Dialectical behavior therapy, often in group classes, teaches a wide range of skills for self-management of emotions and for maintaining the ability to think and problem-solve even in the presence of strong emotions. Yoga, meditation, support groups, religious organizations, and social activities are all of some use, and physicians should recommend these community resources when they are available.

Self-management applies to physicians and patients. When dealing with difficult relationships, the support and advice of colleagues (either informally or through structured interaction, such as a Balint group) is essential, and should be sought out regularly. More formal supervision or personal therapy can be useful.

SUMMARY/DISCUSSION

Primary care physicians often evaluate and treat personality-disordered people in the context of other medical problems. The focus in such care is not the personality disorder per se, but the doctor-patient relationship. Evaluation is appropriately focused on how the relationship is going and on how doctor and patient are collaborating on overall health care. Importantly, the primary care physician can affirm relationship progress and the doctor's office can be a place to make commitments about next steps in overcoming problematic personality traits. This involves constant adjustments to each party's expectations of the other. Recurrence of problematic patterns is to be expected at times of increased stress, and should be addressed with patience and good will. As one author[7] puts it, "A core strategy for family physicians is an intervention based on active listening, mindfulness, and strengthening the connection to the patient's most cherished values."

REFERENCES

1. Bender DS, Dolan RT, Skodol AE, et al. Treatment utilization by patients with personality disorders. Am J Psychiatry 2001;158(2):295–302.
2. Bienenfeld D. Personality disorders treatment & management. In: Ahmed I, editor. Medscape drugs & diseases. New York: Medscape; 2013. Available at: http://emedicine.medscape.com/article/294307-treatment. Accessed August 10, 2015.
3. American Psychiatric Association. Diagnostic and statistical manual of mental disorders. 5th edition. Arlington (VA): American Psychiatric Publishing; 2013.
4. Tyrer P, Coombs N, Ibrahimi F, et al. Critical developments in the assessment of personality disorder. Br J Psychiatry Suppl 2007;190(Suppl 49):s51–9.
5. Silk KR. Caught in an unconscious split: commentary on "the ironic fate of the personality disorders in DSM-5". Personal Disord 2013;4(4):350–1.
6. Cannarella Lorenzetti R, Jacques CH, Donovan C, et al. Managing difficult encounters: understanding physician, patient, and situational factors. Am Fam Physician 2013;87(6):419–25.
7. Stanley JC. Physicians and the difficult patient. Soc Work 1991;36:71–9.
8. King-Casas B, Sharp C, Lomax-Bream L, et al. The rupture and repair of cooperation in borderline personality disorder. Science 2008;321:806–10.
9. National Health and Medical Research Council. Clinical practice guideline for the management of borderline personality disorder. Melbourne (Australia): National Health and Medical Research Council; 2012.
10. Bateman AW, Gunderson J, Mulder R. Treatment of personality disorder. Lancet 2015;385:735–43.
11. Silk KR. Personality disorders. In: Skodol A, editor. UpToDate. Waltham (MA): UpToDate; 2016. Available at: http://www.uptodate.com/contents/personality-disorders?source=machineLearning&search=personality+disorders&selectedTitle=1%7E150&sectionRank=1&anchor=H256373449#H1. Accessed August 10, 2015.
12. Angstman KB, Rasmussen NH. Personality disorders: review and clinical application in daily practice. Am Fam Physician 2011;84(11):1253–60.
13. Ward RK. Assessment and management of personality disorders. Am Fam Physician 2004;70(8):1505–12.
14. Stoffers JM, Völlm BA, Rücker G, et al. Psychological therapies for people with borderline personality disorder. Cochrane Database Syst Rev 2012;(8):CD005652.

Bipolar Disorder

Thomas H. Miller, MD

KEYWORDS

• Bipolar disorder • Manic • Mood stabilizers • Lithium

KEY POINTS

- One in 5 primary care patients who have clinically significant depressive symptoms and are receiving treatment actually have bipolar 1 or 2 disorder.
- Accurate diagnosis and long-term treatment are critical in improving functioning.
- Antidepressant monotherapy is contraindicated in bipolar disorder.
- Primary care physicians should be aware of comorbidities in patients with bipolar disorder, such as cardiovascular disease, diabetes, substance abuse, and tobacco use.
- If primary care providers are not comfortable with the diagnosis or management of bipolar disorder, referral to a mental health specialist is mandatory.

INTRODUCTION

Bipolar disorder is a common, complex, and recurrent severe mental health condition with progressive social and cognitive function disturbances and comorbid medical problems. Estimated to affect 1.5% of the population,[1] bipolar disorder has a typical onset between 13 and 30 years of age and is usually diagnosed after years of symptoms. Bipolar is characterized by mania or hypomania with overactivity, disinhibited behavior, and elation, interspersed with episodes of depression characterized by profound loss of motivation and interest. In primary care, individuals typically do not present with hypomania, rather they present with depressive symptoms. Estimates are that up to 20% to 30% of patients seen in primary care settings for depressive and/or anxiety symptoms actually have bipolar disorder,[2] and up to two-thirds of patients with bipolar disorder can experience other mental health disorders such as anxiety, substance misuse, or impulse-control disorders.[1] Patients with bipolar disorder die earlier than the general population,[3] with increased risk of suicide, unintentional injury, and physical illness, such as ischemic heart disease, diabetes, chronic obstructive lung disease, and pneumonia. Accurate diagnosis and management of this condition is critical for the long-term care of these patients while decreasing attendant morbidity.

Disclosure: The author indicates that he has no commercial or financial conflict of interest.
SIU Quincy Family Medicine Residency, Clinical Family and Community Medicine, SIU School of Medicine, 612 North 11th Street, Quincy, IL 62301, USA
E-mail address: tmiller1@siumed.edu

Prim Care Clin Office Pract 43 (2016) 269–284
http://dx.doi.org/10.1016/j.pop.2016.02.003   **primarycare.theclinics.com**
0095-4543/16/$ – see front matter © 2016 Elsevier Inc. All rights reserved.

SCREENING AND DIAGNOSIS

Bipolar disorder is common and often unrecognized in primary care. As many as 30% of primary care patients seen for depression and or anxiety symptoms may have bipolar disorder. Because patients with bipolar disorder often seek treatment when they are depressed, primary care providers should be aware of the signs and symptoms so as to diagnose bipolar disorder. **Fig. 1** reveals an algorithm for approaching the patient with depression symptoms.[2] The essential feature in making a diagnosis of bipolar disorder is the presence of a manic or hypomanic episode.

Mania and hypomania are similar in that each requires an abnormal, distinct, and persistent increase in energy, accompanied by an elevated and expansive or irritable mood. The 2 differ in their severity, duration, and number of symptoms. Symptoms common to both include the need for less sleep, the presence of pressured speech with flight of ideas, and an involvement in activities with high potential for adverse outcomes.[14] Bipolar 1 disorder requires a manic episode, whereas bipolar 2 disorder requires a hypomanic episode and current or past major depression. The differentiation between a manic and hypomanic episode is based on the number of days of symptoms: 7 versus 4, as well as the degree of impairment in work, family, and social functioning. Hospitalization and psychosis represent such a degree of impairment that these situations are only attributed to bipolar 1. The DSM-5 diagnostic criteria for Bipolar Disorder can be found in the DSM-5.[14]

Two different tools that are helpful in the diagnosis of bipolar disorder include the mood disorder questionnaire (MDQ) and the Composite International Diagnostic Interview 3 (CIDI 3.0) (**Tables 1** and **2**). The MDQ is a patient self-reported instrument that has 3 questions. The first asks about 13 different life situations or occurrences. The events that are described are very similar to the diagnostic criteria from the *Diagnostic and Statistical Manual of Mental Disorders, Fifth Edition* (DSM-5), which are summarized in. The second question asks if more than 1 of the 13 situations occurred simultaneously. And, the third, defines the degree of effect on social functioning. A positive screen occurs when the patient lists at least 7 of 13 symptom items, confirms that 2 or more symptoms occurred simultaneously, and indicates that his or her functional impairment due to symptoms was moderate or worse.[2]

The World Mental Health Organization CIDI 3.0 is designed to be used in a brief structured clinical interview (**Table 2**). The stem items ask about the patient experiencing extreme euphoria or an abnormally irritable mood. If the patient answers the stem questions affirmatively, then a series of screening and symptom questions follow. Once again, the 9 situations, events, and impressions are similar to the DSM-5 diagnostic criteria. If the first 2 stem questions are denied, no additional questions are needed. These 2 tools use common language and easy-to-understand events and impressions to respectively help the patient or medical professional evaluate for the presence or absence of mania or hypomania. The MDQ also directly assesses the degree of functional impairment associated with a manic or hypomanic episode. Use of these 2 rating systems may help with the diagnosis. Confirmation with both screening tools, in addition to the clinical interview, may lend diagnostic support, whereas conflicting information may justify consultation or referral.

Substance abuse, medication-related effects, and a number of medical problems can lead to manic or hypomanic behavior (**Box 1**). The drugs of abuse include classic agents that would cause accelerated mood or irritability, as well as some not always suspected of causing these behaviors. Beyond drugs of abuse, legally prescribed

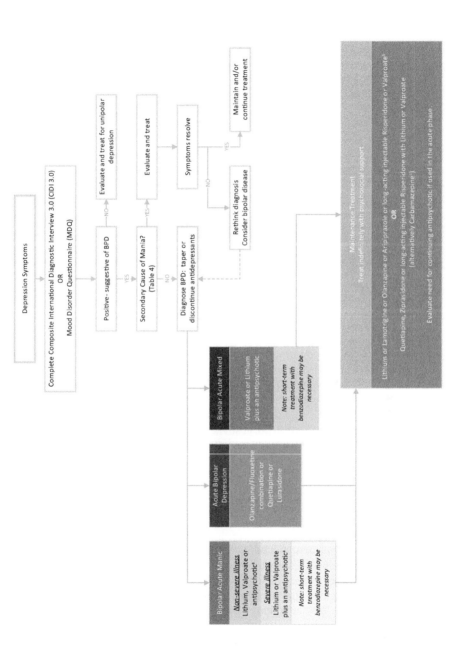

Fig. 1. Depression symptom algorithm. [a] Atypical antipsychotics are preferred over typical antipsychotics. Best evidence: olanzapine and risperidone.[16] [b] Not FDA approved for maintenance but frequently used. [c] Oxcarbazepine may have better tolerability and equivalent efficacy than carbamazepine. Less evidence. (*Data from* Refs. [1,4–13])

Table 1
Mood disorder questionnaire to be used as a patient self-reported instrument

		YES	NO
1.	Has there ever been a period of time when you were not your usual self and…		
	You felt so good or so hyper that other people thought you were not your normal self or you were so hyper that you got into trouble?	☐	☐
	You were so irritable that you shouted at people or started fights or arguments?	☐	☐
	You felt much more self-confident than usual?	☐	☐
	You got much less sleep than usual and found you didn't really miss it?	☐	☐
	You were much more talkative or spoke faster than usual?	☐	☐
	Thoughts raced through your head or you couldn't slow your mind down?	☐	☐
	You were so easily distracted by things around you that you had trouble concentrating or staying on track?	☐	☐
	You had much more energy than usual?	☐	☐
	You were much more active or did many more things than usual?	☐	☐
	You were much more social or outgoing than usual, for example, you telephoned friends in the middle of the night?	☐	☐
	You were much more interested in sex than usual?	☐	☐
	You did things that were unusual for you or that other people might have thought were excessive, foolish, or risky?	☐	☐
	Spending money got you or your family into trouble?	☐	☐
2.	If you checked YES to more than 1 of the above, have several of these ever happened during the same period of time? *Please circle one response only* YES NO		
3.	How much of a problem did any of these cause you, such as being unable to work; having family, money, or legal troubles; getting into arguments or fights? *Please circle one response only* *No Problem Minor Problem Moderate Problem Serious Problem*		

From Hirschfeld RMA, Bowden CL, Gitlin MJ, et al. Practice guideline for the treatment of patients with bipolar disorder. 2nd edition. American Psychiatric Association; 2010; ©2000 by Robert M.A. Hirschfeld, MD. Reprinted with permission.

medications can also cause secondary mania. The medication categories include cardiovascular, endocrine, psychiatric, and other assorted agents. Importantly, antidepressant monotherapy can trigger a manic or hypomanic episode. Offending agents should be discontinued or, if not possible, reduced to the lowest dosage.

Medical problems that could mimic or exacerbate manic or hypomanic episodes should be identified. The primary care provider is in an excellent position to diagnose these conditions. Particular attention should be focused on collagen vascular diseases, endocrine disorders, infectious diseases, neurologic syndromes, and nutritional deficiencies. A complete history and physical examination and standard chemistry, hematologic, and thyroid laboratory panels should be obtained. Targeted additional laboratory, cardiac, imaging, or neurologic function testing should be performed based on the results of the history and physical examination, as needed to diagnose or rule out conditions that could cause or exacerbate a manic or hypomanic episode (**Table 3**).

Table 2
Questions used in the CIDI-based bipolar disorder screening scale

I. Stem questions

1. Some people have periods lasting several days or longer when they feel much more excited and full of energy than usual. Their minds go too fast. They talk a lot. They are very restless or unable to sit still and they sometimes do things that are unusual for them, such as driving too fast or spending too much money. Have you ever had a period like this lasting several days or longer?[a]

2. Have you ever had a period lasting several days or longer when most of the time you were so irritable or grouchy that you either started arguments, shouted at people, or hit people?

II. Criterion B screening question

1. People who have episodes like this often have changes in their thinking and behavior at the same time, like being more talkative, needing very little sleep, being very restless, going on buying sprees, and behaving in ways they would normally think are inappropriate. Did you ever have any of these changes during your episodes of being (excited and full of energy/ very irritable or grouchy)?

III. Criterion B symptom questions

Think of an episode when you had the largest number of changes like these at the same time. During that episode, which of the following changes did you experience?

1. Were you so irritable that you either started arguments, shouted at people, or hit people?[b]

2. Did you become so restless or fidgety that you paced up and down or couldn't stand still?

3. Did you do anything else that wasn't usual for you, like talking about things you would normally keep private, or acting in ways that you'd usually find embarrassing?

4. Did you try to do things that were impossible to do, like taking on large amounts of work?

5. Did you constantly keep changing your plans or activities?

6. Did you find it hard to keep your mind on what you were doing?

7. Did your thoughts seem to jump from one thing to another or race through your head so fast you couldn't keep track of them?

8. Did you sleep far less than usual and still not get tired or sleepy?

9. Did you spend so much more money than usual that it caused you to have financial trouble?

Abbreviation: CIDI, Composite International Diagnostic Interview.
    [a] If this question is endorsed, the irritability stem question is skipped and the respondent goes directly to the Criterion B screening question.
    [b] This question is asked only if the euphoria stem question is endorsed.
From Kessler RC, Akiskal HS, Angst J, et al. Validity of the assessment of bipolar spectrum disorders in the WHO CIDI 3.0. J Affect Disord 2006;96(3):259–69. © 2013 World Health Organization. All rights reserved. Used with permission.

MANAGEMENT AND GOALS

The following points are crucial in managing the patient with bipolar disorder:

1. Establish an accurate diagnosis of bipolar disorder and type.
2. Rule out medical conditions and substance abuse, which can mimic manic and depressive symptoms.[3,15]
3. Determine the optimum treatment location by considering the patient's safety and level of functioning.[4] Hospitalization is necessary if the patient is a threat to self or others.
4. Avoid mono therapy with antidepressants as contraindicated.
5. Treat bipolar disorder to decrease morbidity and mortality. Ongoing therapy is needed, as there is no cure.

Box 1
Selected causes of secondary mania

Drug abuse

Alcohol, amphetamines, cocaine, hallucinogens, opiates

Medications

Cardiovascular: captopril, hydralazine

Endocrine: bromocriptine (Parlodel), corticosteroids

Neurologic agents: levodopa

Psychiatric: antidepressants, disulfiram (Antabuse), methylphenidate (Ritalin), monoamine oxidase inhibitors

Other agents: baclofen (Lioresal), cimetidine (Tagamet), isoniazid

Diseases

Collagen vascular disease: systemic lupus erythematosus

Endocrine disease: Cushing disease, hyperthyroidism or hypothyroidism

Infectious disease: herpes encephalitis, human immunodeficiency virus encephalitis, influenza, neurosyphilis

Neurologic disease: complex partial seizures, Huntington chorea, migraine headache, multiple sclerosis, neoplasm, stroke, traumatic brain injury, Wilson disease

Vitamin deficiency: B_{12}, folate, niacin, thiamine

From Family Practice Notebook. Available at: http://www.fpnotebook.com/. Accessed August 19, 2015; with permission; and *Data from* Price AL, Marzani-Nissen GR. Bipolar disorders: a review. Am Fam Physician 2012;85(5):483–93; and Werder SF. An update on the diagnosis and treatment of mania in bipolar disorder. Am Fam Physician 1995;51(5):1126–36.

---

6. Establish a therapeutic alliance: monitor the patient's psychiatric and functional status, provide education, and ensure treatment compliance.
7. Promote regular patterns of activity and of sleep, anticipate stressors, and identify new episodes early to minimize functional impairment.[5,16]
8. Stabilize the acute episode with a goal of returning to baseline level of function and a virtual lack of symptoms.
9. Use the patient-specific combination of pharmacologic, self-management, and nonpharmacologic therapies.
10. Protect against recurrence of depressive mixed, manic, or hypomanic episodes.
11. Maximize patient functioning and minimize subthreshold symptoms and adverse effects of treatment.[4]
12. Beware of comorbidities, such as cardiovascular disease, diabetes, chronic obstructive pulmonary disease, influenza or pneumonia, unintentional injuries, and suicide.[17]

PHARMACOLOGIC STRATEGIES

After an accurate diagnosis is made, pharmacologic therapy is considered. **Table 4** outlines preferred medications for each instance, as well as tips on titration or augmentation. Of note again, monotherapy with an antidepressant not only lacks

Table 3
Medical tests to consider in the evaluation of patients with a suspected bipolar disorder

Test	Rationale
Basic metabolic panel, more detailed evaluation of renal function (in patients with a history of renal disease)	Establishes baseline sodium level and renal function in patients taking antipsychotics, lithium, anticonvulsants, and antidepressants
Complete blood count	Rules out pernicious anemia, establishes baseline measurements in patients taking anticonvulsants
Complete physical examination, including neurologic evaluation	May help rule out systemic illness; establishes baseline measurements of body mass index, blood pressure, and waist circumference, which are monitored in maintenance treatment of bipolar disorders; routine maintenance examination includes monitoring for medication adverse effects, including extrapyramidal effects
Electrocardiography (in patients older than 40 y, in others if indicated)	Establishes baseline measurements in patients taking lithium, antipsychotics, or medications that can prolong the QTc interval (nonpsychiatric medications, such as proton pump inhibitors, carbamazepine [Tegretol], and prochlorperazine)
Fasting glucose level, lipid profile	Rules out diabetes mellitus, hyperlipidemia, and Cushing syndrome and establishes baseline measurements in patients taking any medication that can cause weight gain or hyperglycemia
Liver function tests, prothrombin time, and partial thromboplastin time (if electroconvulsive therapy is planned)	May help rule out hepatitis, establishes baseline measurements in patients taking anticonvulsants and antipsychotics
Pregnancy test (if relevant)	Avoids use of teratogenic medications in pregnancy
Prolactin level	Establishes baseline measurements in patients taking antipsychotics, which increase prolactin level
Thyroid-stimulating hormone level	Rules out primary or secondary thyroid disorders, establishes baseline measurements in patients taking lithium
Urinalysis	Helps rule out infection in older patients
Urine toxicology screen	Rules out mood and thought disorders secondary to substance abuse
Additional tests in patient with new-onset psychosis Electroencephalography MRI (preferred) or computed tomography If indicated based on clinical suspicion: urine toxicology and studies for heavy metals, urine porphyrins, hepatitis C, and syphilis	Rules out occult seizure disorder, intracranial mass, other causes of secondary psychosis

From Price AL, Marzani-Nissen GR. Bipolar disorders: a review. Am Fam Physician 2012;85(5): 483–93; with permission.

Table 4
Pharmacologic management of bipolar disorder

Medication	Problem	Management
None	Acute bipolar depression	Start OFC, quetiapine, or lurasidone
OFC or quetiapine or lurasidone	No response to bipolar moderate-severe depression	Add lamotrigine
Lamotrigine	Inadequate response in bipolar depression	Increase dose, if at maximum add lithium
Lithium	Moderate-severe bipolar depression	If inadequate level, supplement. If adequate dose, add OFC or quetiapine; or add olanzapine (without fluoxetine) or lamotrigine
Lithium and OFC or lithium and quetiapine	Inadequate response	Stop OFC and quetiapine and add lamotrigine to lithium
Lithium or valproate plus an antipsychotic	Acute bipolar manic or mixed, inadequate response	Optimize doses. If optimal doses, add additional mood stabilizer. Alternatively, add carbamazepine or oxcarbamazepine; or change antipsychotic
None	Maintenance therapy with mania prevention preference	Lithium or long-acting injectable risperidone or olanzapine or aripiprazole
None	Maintenance therapy with depression prevention preference	Lamotrigine or quetiapine. Quetiapine with lithium or valproate
Maximum medical therapy	Acute bipolar manic or mixed	Consider change of antipsychotic for clozapine or refer for right unilateral electroconvulsive therapy

Abbreviation: OFC, olanzapine/fluoxetine combination.
Data from Refs.[1,5,6,9,18–20]

efficacy in the acute treatment of bipolar depression but may also worsen the long-term course of the illness. For acute bipolar depression, 3 therapeutic options approved by the Food and Drug Administration (FDA) are available: olanzapine/fluoxetine combination, quetiapine or lurasidone monotherapy (see **Fig. 1**). The number needed to treat in placebo-controlled trials for each of these agents is similar. When considering pharmacologic options for treatment, the clinician should take advantage of known medication side effects. For example, if the patient and/or clinician feel that some degree of sedation can be helpful with anxiety during the day and for sleep in the evening, then an agent with that side-effect profile may remove the need for additional medications. The experience of the clinician, as well as the history of tolerability and efficacy of particular agents in the individual patient, must be considered in choosing a medication. For acute bipolar, manic or mixed, the options include lithium or valproate plus an antipsychotic.[5] Five mono therapies and 3 combination therapies are approved for the longer-term treatment of bipolar disorder.

Table 5 outlines the medication choices for treatment of bipolar disorders and their specific indications. In addition, **Table 6** lists specific dosing recommendations, side

Table 5
Medication therapy for patients with bipolar disorders

Medication	Indication			Comments
	Acute Mania	Maintenance	Acute Bipolar Depression	
Antipsychotics, atypical	—	—	—	Antipsychotic medication plus lithium or an anticonvulsant is superior to monotherapy for acute mania
Aripiprazole (Abilify)	Yes[ab]	Yes[a]	No	—
Olanzapine (Zyprexa)	Yes[ab]	Yes[a]	Yes (plus SSRI)[a]	Olanzapine and aripiprazole are effective in preventing manic relapse
Quetiapine (Seroquel)	Yes[a]	Yes[a]	Yes[a]	Quetiapine plus lithium or valproate is superior to monotherapy for maintenance treatment
Risperidone (Risperdal)	Yes[ab]	Yes[a]	No	—
Ziprasidone (Geodon)	Yes[a]	Yes[a]	No	—
Asenapine (Saphris)	Yes[ab]	No	No	—
Lurasidone (Latuda)	No	No	Yes[a]	—
Antipsychotics, typical				
Haloperidol lactate (Haldol)	Yes	No	No	No difference in response rates among haloperidol, risperidone, olanzapine, carbamazepine, and valproate for acute mania
Benzodiazepines				
Lorazepam (Ativan)	Yes	No	No	Used as combination therapy in patients with acute mania to reduce agitation
Carbamazepine (Tegretol)	Yes[a]	Yes	Yes	Evidence for carbamazepine is not as strong as that for lithium and valproate
Divalproex (Depakote), valproic acid (Depakene)	Yes[a]	Yes	Yes	Valproate appears to be more effective than lithium for mixed states
Lamotrigine (Lamictal)	No	Yes[a]	Yes	Acceptable agent in pregnancy; associated with weight loss in obese patients with bipolar 1 disorder
Lithium	Yes[a]	Yes[a]	Yes	Lithium lowers suicide risk compared with valproate or carbamazepine. Lithium appears to be protective against dementia[15]. Adding an SSRI or bupropion (Wellbutrin) does not improve depressive symptoms

Abbreviation: SSRI, selective serotonin reuptake inhibitor.

[a] Approved by the Food and Drug Administration.

[b] Approved monotherapy or in combination with lithium, valproate, or carbamazepine.

Data from Price AL, Marzani-Nissen GR. Bipolar disorders: a review. Am Fam Physician 2012;85(5):483–93.

Table 6
Dosing and monitoring of medications for bipolar disorders

Medication	Dosing Information	Common Adverse Effects	Monitoring Recommendations	Comments
Antipsychotics, atypical Aripiprazole (Abilify) Olanzapine (Zyprexa) Quetiapine (Seroquel) Risperidone (Risperdal) Ziprasidone (Geodon) Asenapine (Saphris) Lurasidone (Sunovion)	Varies	Somnolence, dry mouth, orthostatic hypotension, extrapyramidal effects, akathisia, tardive dyskinesia, weight gain, hyperglycemia, neuroleptic malignant syndrome, hyperprolactinemia, sexual dysfunction	Lipid profile, fasting blood glucose level, waist circumference, body weight, and CBC in patients with prior clinically significant leukopenia; measure at baseline, monthly in the first 3 mo of therapy, then every 3 mo thereafter	Quetiapine, risperidone, and ziprasidone increase the risk of extrapyramidal effects Ziprasidone, lurasidone, and aripiprazole cause less weight gain and hyperlipidemia Caution should be used when decreasing dosages because rebound anxiety and psychosis are possible Increased risk of death in older patients with dementia[a]
Antipsychotics, typical Haloperidol lactate (Haldol)	2–5 mg intramuscularly for acute episode; may repeat every hour as needed until symptoms are controlled; switch to oral form as soon as feasible Initial dosage is based on patient's age and severity of symptoms; dosage rarely should exceed 100 mg in 24 hours No recommendation for use after acute episode	Insomnia, restlessness, anxiety, sedation, headache, seizures, weight gain, psychosis, hypotension, tardive dyskinesia, extrapyramidal effects, depression, QT prolongation, neuroleptic malignant syndrome, pneumonia, blood dyscrasia, hyperprolactinemia	CBC (in patients with prior clinically significant leukopenia) at baseline and monthly in the first 3 mo of therapy Prolactin level as clinically indicated Monitor for extrapyramidal effects, tardive dyskinesia, and neuroleptic malignant syndrome	Increased risk of death in older patients with dementia[a] Torsades de pointes possible, particularly with higher than recommended dosages

Drug	Dosage	Adverse effects	Monitoring	Precautions
Benzodiazepines Lorazepam (Ativan)	0.5–2.0 mg orally or intramuscularly, up to 4.0 mg per day Reduce dose by 50% in patients who are older and debilitated, patients taking valproate, and patients with hepatic or renal disease	Sedation, nausea, blood dyscrasia, extrapyramidal effects, agitation, anterograde amnesia, cognitive impairment, respiratory depression, hyponatremia, syndrome of inappropriate antidiuretic hormone	Periodic CBC and liver function testing for patients on long-term therapy	Contraindicated in patients with myasthenia gravis or acute narrow-angle glaucoma Avoid in patients with history of substance abuse Continuous long-term use not recommended Paradoxic reactions are more likely in children and older persons; risk of seizure after discontinuation is greater in patients with preexisting seizure disorder and in those taking antidepressants
Carbamazepine (Tegretol)	200–1600 mg orally per day Begin with 200 mg twice per day, adjusting every day by 200 mg as tolerated Titrate to serum level of 4–12 μg per mL	Headache; fatigue; nystagmus; ataxia; rash, including Stevens-Johnson syndrome and toxic epidermal necrolysis[a]; leukopenia, hyponatremia	Serum carbamazepine levels every 1 to 2 wk initially, then every 3 to 6 mo or before and after dosage changes CBC and liver function testing monthly for the first 2 mo, then every 3 to 12 mo thereafter Screening for HLA-B1502 in patients with Asian ancestry; patients with positive screening results should avoid carbamazepine because of the risk of Stevens-Johnson syndrome and toxic epidermal necrolysis	Slower titration mitigates adverse effects Hyponatremia occurs in up to 40% of patients

(continued on next page)

Table 6
(continued)

Medication	Dosing Information	Common Adverse Effects	Monitoring Recommendations	Comments
Oxcarbazepine (Trileptal)	Target dosage: 1200 mg per day Begin with 300 mg orally bid Increase by 300 mg per day every 3 d or by 600 mg per day every week	Abdominal pain, nausea, diplopia, abnormal gait, dizziness, vertigo, somnolence, tremor, rash including Stevens-Johnson syndrome and toxic epidermal necrolysis	May lower serum sodium, monitor 2–4 wk during initiation and periodically during maintenance, especially if prescribed with other medications that could lower serum sodium 25%–30% chance of hypersensitivity if reaction to carbamazepine. Consider screening for *HLA-B1502* in patients with Asian ancestry; patients with positive screening results should avoid oxcarbazepine because of the risk of Stevens-Johnson syndrome and toxic epidermal necrolysis	If creatinine clearance <30, start at 300 mg per day. Pregnancy Category C
Divalproex (Depakote), valproic acid (Depakene)	Target dosage: 1000–3000 mg orally per day 15–20 mg per kg load in patients with acute mania; may also start with 500–750 mg per day in divided doses and adjust every 2 to 3 days as tolerated Titrate to serum level of 50–125 µg per mL	Tremor, sedation, weight gain, nausea, diarrhea, hair loss, leukopenia, thrombocytopenia, elevated liver transaminase levels, hepatic failure,[a] pancreatitis,[a] polycystic ovary syndrome	Serum valproate levels every 1 to 2 wk initially, then every 3 to 6 mo or before and after dosage changes CBC and liver function testing monthly for the first 2 mo, then every 3 to 12 mo thereafter	Polycystic ovary syndrome is common in women who start treatment before 20 y of age Teratogenic[a]

Lamotrigine (Lamictal)	200 mg orally per day Begin with 25 mg per day, and titrate over 6 wk; titration and dosage adjustments differ for those taking valproic acid, carbamazepine, phenytoin (Dilantin), phenobarbital, primidone (Mysoline), rifampin, and oral contraceptives	Dizziness; tremor; somnolence; headache; dry mouth; nausea; rash, including Stevens-Johnson syndrome and toxic epidermal necrolysis[a]; leukopenia; thrombocytopenia; pancytopenia; aseptic meningitis	CBC and liver function testing monthly for the first 2 mo, then every 3 to 12 mo thereafter	The incidence of skin rash is reduced with slow titration and by not exceeding the recommended dosage Incidence of serious rash in adults is 0.08% with monotherapy
Lithium	900–1800 mg orally per day Begin with up to 300 mg twice per day, and adjust dosage every 2 or 3 d as tolerated; titrate to serum level of 0.6–1.5 mEq per L	Thirst, polyuria, cognitive effects, sedation, tremor, weight gain, diarrhea, nausea, hypothyroidism, diabetes insipidus	Serum lithium levels every 1 to 2 wk initially, then every 3 to 6 mo thereafter or before and after dosage changes Thyroid function testing[b] and renal indices every 2 or 3 mo in the first 6 mo of therapy, then every 6 to 12 mo thereafter	Toxicity is dose dependent; overdose can be fatal[a] Incidence of hypothyroidism is higher in women and increases with age High rates of withdrawal compared with valproate and lamotrigine in maintenance therapy

Abbreviation: CBC, complete blood count.

[a] US Food and Drug Administration boxed warning.

[b] Thyroid-stimulating hormone, total thyroxine, thyroxine uptake.

Data from Price AL, Marzani-Nissen GR. Bipolar disorders: a review. Am Fam Physician 2012;85(5):483–93; and Drugs for psychiatric disorders. Treat Guidel Med Lett 2013;11(13):53–64.

effects, and appropriate monitoring to be undertaken with each medication prescribed. If the primary care provider is with or lacks experience or knowledge in prescribing approved medications, the patient should be referred to a mental health specialist.

NONPHARMACOLOGIC STRATEGIES

A key part of treatment of bipolar includes helping the patient and the patient's support system understand the disorder itself. The clinician should provide individuals with information about bipolar disorder: its treatment, diagnosis, symptoms, and medication management. Combined with pharmacotherapy, psychoeducational, family, cognitive behavioral therapy (CBT), and interpersonal therapies have been used to improve function and decrease the likelihood and severity of future episodes. Programs that teach early recognition of signs and symptoms of impending manic or depressive episodes have been shown to decrease time to first recurrence. Psychoeducational interventions succeeded in improving overall function and lowering the percentage of people hospitalized.[16]

Family-intervention goals include accepting the reality of the illness and its long-term treatment, identifying and strategizing on how to minimize or remove future stressors, and elucidating familial interactions that may put stress on the patient. Family-focused therapy that includes education, communication training, and problem-solving skills therapy resulted in lower depression relapse and improved pharmacologic adherence.[9]

CBT programs educate the patient regarding bipolar disorder and its treatment, teach skills for coping with psychological stressors, facilitate medication compliance, and monitor the occurrence and severity of symptoms. In patients with refractory bipolar disorder, CBT with pharmacotherapy resulted in less hospitalization, lower depression and anxiety, less mania, and improved social-occupational function.[21]

Interpersonal and social rhythm therapy reduces depressive symptoms, and manic and hypomanic episodes, and results in more euthymic days. This type of therapy incorporates behavioral self-monitoring to maintain a lifestyle of regular sleep-wake cycles, meal times, physical activity, and emotional stimulation.[4]

SELF-MANAGEMENT STRATEGIES

The individual plays a central role in bipolar management.[22] Goals of self-management are to provide individuals with needed knowledge and skills to participate actively in their health care. Self-management should complement and not replace psychotherapeutic care for bipolar disorder. Many partner management delivery modalities are available. Strategies include the use of workbooks, mobile technologies, and Internet-based or peer-led interventions. The areas that should be covered overlap and include the following:

1. Providing education on accurate diagnosis, symptoms, medication adherence, and side effects, and avoidance of substance use.
2. Self-monitoring mood, depression, and energy daily.
3. Optimizing sleep hygiene.
4. Setting goals in the following domains: relationships, employment, education, health, recreation, house/homecare, and self-management.
5. Prioritizing healthy lifestyle: regular physical activity, healthy eating, and weight loss and/or weight management.[23,24]

EVALUATION ADJUSTMENT RECURRENCE

One of the hallmarks of bipolar disorder is that it is a chronic illness characterized by recurrence. Subsequent to each episode of mania or bipolar depression, clinicians should discuss the longer-term management plan with the patient and caregivers. Treatment for bipolar disorder is lifelong, and the clinician must consider the tolerability of medications in establishing a long-term management plan. In general, the lowest, most-effective dose should be used. When managing recurrent episodes of mania or bipolar depression, the clinician should be aware of and consider medications that have been successful in the past. Multiple medication combinations may be needed, and if the primary care clinician is not comfortable or knowledgeable about the use of the agents, referral to a more experienced clinician is mandatory (**Table 4**). Self-management and nonpharmacologic strategies, as outlined previously, that include group, family, or individual psychological therapy designed for bipolar disorder have some evidence in preventing relapse and in helping those with persistent symptoms between episodes of mania or bipolar depression.

SUMMARY/DISCUSSION

Patients who present to primary care physicians with depressive symptoms should be screened for the presence of several days or longer of mania or extreme irritability. Several conditions can mimic or cause bipolar disorder, and these should be ruled out by history, physical examination, and directed testing. Pharmacologic treatment of bipolar disorder is lifelong. Treatment for bipolar disorder with antidepressant monotherapy is contraindicated. The primary care provider should be aware of the indications, side effects, and dosages of appropriate pharmacologic therapy or refer the patient. Patients with bipolar disorder should be monitored for the development of comorbidities, including cardiovascular and metabolic disorders. Nonpharmacologic interventions, including CBT and self-management strategies, enhance long-term outcomes.

REFERENCES

1. Kendall T, Morriss R, Mayo-Wilson E, et al, on behalf of the Guideline Development Group of the National Institute for Health and Care Excellence. Assessment and management of bipolar disorder: summary of updated NICE guidance. BMJ 2014;349:g5673.

2. Manning JS. Tools to improve differential diagnosis of bipolar disorder in primary care. Prim Care Companion J Clin Psychiatry 2010;12(Suppl 1):17–22.

3. Scrandis DA. Identification and management of bipolar disorder. Nurse Pract 2014;39(10):30–7 [quiz: 37–8].

4. Hirschfeld RMA, Bowden CL, Gitlin MJ, et al. Practice guideline for the treatment of patients with bipolar disorder. 2nd edition. American Psychiatric Association; 2010.

5. Citrome L. Treatment of bipolar depression: making sensible decisions. CNS Spectr 2014;19(Suppl 1):4–11 [quiz: 1–3, 12].

6. Post RM, Ostacher MJ, Singh V. Controversies in the psychopharmacology of bipolar disorder. J Clin Psychiatry 2014;75(11):e30.

7. Nierenberg AA. A critical appraisal of treatments for bipolar disorder. Prim Care Companion J Clin Psychiatry 2010;12(Suppl 1):23–9.

8. Cipriani A, Reid K, Young AH, et al. Valproic acid, valproate and divalproex in the maintenance treatment of bipolar disorder. Cochrane Database Syst Rev 2013;(10):CD003196.
9. Burgess SS, Geddes J, Hawton KK, et al. Lithium for maintenance treatment of mood disorders. Cochrane Database Syst Rev 2001;(3):CD003013.
10. Cipriani A, Rendell JM, Geddes J. Haloperidol alone or in combination for acute mania. Cochrane Database Syst Rev 2006;(3):CD004362.
11. Rendell JM, Gijsman HJ, Bauer MS, et al. Risperidone alone or in combination for acute mania. Cochrane Database Syst Rev 2006;(1):CD004043.
12. Vasudev A, Macritchie K, Vasudev K, et al. Oxcarbazepine for acute affective episodes in bipolar disorder. Cochrane Database Syst Rev 2011;(12):CD004857.
13. Vasudev A, Macritchie K, Watson S, et al. Oxcarbazepine in the maintenance of bipolar disorder. Cochrane Database Syst Rev 2008;(1):CD005171.
14. American Psychiatric Association. Bipolar disorder. In: Diagnostic and statistical manual of mental disorders. 5th edition. Washington, DC: American Psychiatric Publishing; 2013. p. 124–5.
15. Price AL, Marzani-Nissen GR. Bipolar disorders: a review. Am Fam Physician 2012;85(5):483–93.
16. Morriss R, Faizal MA, Jones AP, et al. Interventions for helping people recognize early signs of recurrence in bipolar disorder. Cochrane Database Syst Rev 2007;(1):CD004854.
17. Crump C, Sundquist K, Winkleby MA, et al. Comorbidities and mortality in bipolar disorder: a Swedish National Cohort Study. JAMA Psychiatry 2013;70(9):931–9.
18. Gallagher P, Malik N, Newham J, et al. Antiglucocorticoid treatments for mood disorders. Cochrane Database Syst Rev 2008;(1):CD005168.
19. Rendell JM, Geddes J. Risperidone in long-term treatment for bipolar disorder. Cochrane Database Syst Rev 2006;(4):CD004999.
20. Kessler U, Schoeyen HK, Andreassen OA, et al. The effect of electroconvulsive therapy on neurocognitive function in treatment-resistant bipolar disorder depression. J Clin Psychiatry 2014;75(11):e1306–13.
21. Isasi AG, Echeburua E, Liminana JM, et al. Psychoeducation and cognitive-behavioral therapy for patients with refractory bipolar disorder: a 5-year controlled clinical trial. Eur Psychiatry 2014;29:134–41.
22. Janney CA, Bauer MS, Kilbourne AM. Self-management and bipolar disorder–a clinician's guide to the literature 2011-2014. Curr Psychiatry Rep 2014;16:485.
23. Stoll AL, Severus E, Freeman MP, et al. Omega 3 fatty acids in bipolar disorder: a preliminary double-blind, placebo-controlled trial. Arch Gen Psychiatry 1999;56:407–12.
24. Montgomery P, Richardson AJ. Omega-3 fatty acids for bipolar disorder. Cochrane Database Syst Rev 2008;(2):CD005169.

Autism Spectrum/ Pervasive Developmental Disorder

 CrossMark

Andrew Yochum, DO

KEYWORDS

- Autism spectrum disorder • Primary care physician role
- Comprehensive examination • Autism spectrum disorder–specific screening
- Autism spectrum disorder management

KEY POINTS

- Autism spectrum disorder is characterized by abnormalities in social communication/interaction and restricted, repetitive patterns of behavior, interests, or activities.
- The primary care physician often initiates the workup for the diagnosis of autism spectrum disorder based on both parents' concerns and clinical suspicion from developmental milestone reviews.
- Keep in mind, there is no cure for autism spectrum disorder; however, early diagnosis and early intensive treatment have the potential to affect outcomes in all aspects of the disorder.
- An autism spectrum disorder–specific screening test should be performed anytime autism spectrum disorder concerns are raised during a developmental surveillance. The American Academy of Pediatrics recommends screening at age 18 months and 24 months.
- The overall basis for management of autism spectrum disorder is 3-fold: (1) maximize function, (2) promote a child's independence, and (3) improve quality of life.

INTRODUCTION

What do Curt Schilling—a dominant pitcher, Ernie Els—a masterful golfer, Tommy Hilfiger—a fashionable designer, Toni Braxton—an artistic performer, and Dan Marino—an impeccable quarterback all have in common? The answer: each of their lives has been affected by raising a child who has a pervasive developmental disorder—autism. According to 2010 data from the Autism and Developmental Disabilities Monitoring (ADDM) Network, an estimated 1 in 68 children have an autism

This author does not have any conflict of interest, financially or commercially, as well as any funding to disclose.
Department of Family Medicine, Southern Illinois University-Carbondale, 305 West Jackson Street, Suite 200, Carbondale, IL 62901, USA
E-mail address: ayoch69@gmail.com

spectrum disorder (ASD) diagnosed by the age of 8 years, a marked increase from the 2006 and 2008 estimates of 1 per 111 and 1 per 91, respectively.[1]

The term *autism spectrum disorder* can encompass a broad range in severity from the classic autism behavior to the more highly functional Asperger presentation. However, regardless of location on this neurodevelopmental continuum, ASD is characterized by abnormalities in social communication/interaction and restricted, repetitive patterns of behavior, interests, or activities.[2]

SCREENING/DIAGNOSIS
Terminology and Diagnostic Criteria

The codification and diagnostic criteria of ASD are centered on 2 clinically similar but geographically oriented classification systems: the Diagnostic and Statistical Manual of Mental Disorders (DSM)—predominantly used in the United States—and the World Health Organization International Classification of Diseases, 10th revision (ICD-10)—primarily used by other countries throughout the world.[2,3]

- DSM classification system
  - Updated in May 2013 from DSM-4 to DSM-5
  - Officially termed *autism spectrum disorder* as a single diagnosis encompassing prior DSM-4 disorders of early infantile autism, childhood autism, Kanner's autism, high-functioning autism, atypical autism, pervasive development disorder–not otherwise specified, childhood disintegrative disorder, and Asperger disorder
  - Age requirement
    - No age cutoff; however, must be present in the early childhood development years[2]
- ICD-10 classification system
  - Uses the nomenclature *pervasive developmental disorders*
  - Categorizes into subgroups that include, but are not limited to:
    - Childhood autism
    - Atypical autism
    - Asperger syndrome
    - Pervasive developmental disorder–unspecified
  - Based on 2 sets of guidelines
    - Clinical description and diagnostic guidelines
    - Diagnostic criteria for research
  - Age requirement
    - Symptom onset before age 3[3]

EPIDEMIOLOGY

Approximately 4 times more prevalent in males than females,[4] ASD is a complex entity exhibiting a diverse array of clinical manifestations. As stated earlier, ASD symptoms must be present at some point during the early childhood developmental period, most notably in the 18- to 24-month age range.[5] However, a delayed diagnostic work flow exists that spans, on average, 19 months from the onset of initial symptoms to definitive diagnosis (mean interval of 6 months between onset of parental concern and seeking professional help plus mean interval of 13 months between first documented evaluation and diagnosis).[6,7] Thus, the diagnosis of ASD, on average, occurs at 4.5 years of age.[1]

The nearly 20% higher prevalence rate among siblings of a child with ASD versus the general population,[8] along with a higher concordance rate among monozygotic twins (59%),[9] support the role of genetic factors in the etiology of ASD.[10] Parental age also contributes to an increased prevalence of ASD. Both maternal and paternal age has been shown in multiple research studies to be associated with an increased risk of having a child with ASD. Offspring of a father greater than 40 years old were 5.75 times more likely to have ASD compared with offspring of men younger than 30, possibly because of de novo mutations associated with advancing age.[11] Likewise, the age of expectant mothers has been shown to influence the risk of offspring having ASD. A 2012 meta-analysis supported an independent relationship between higher maternal age and ASD.[12]

A controversial topic in the media over the last few years has been the reported association of ASD with the measles/mumps/rubella (MMR) vaccination. Overwhelmingly, most epidemiologic evidence does not support an association between them. A 2012 retrospective, cohort study reported on the ASD occurrence by MMR vaccine status in US-insured children. Conclusions of this trial showed no evidence that receipt of either 1 or 2 doses of MMR vaccination was associated with an increased risk of ASD among children who had older siblings with ASD or children already at higher risk for ASD.[13]

Epidemiologically, ASD has been associated with specific neurodevelopment conditions[2] such as intellectual disability (45%–60% of ASD patients have some degree of intellectual disability)[14] and seizures (9%–11% prevalence; seizure risk directly correlated to degree of intellectual disability). In addition to these neurologic ailments, ASD has been linked to certain genetic disorders, most commonly[15]:

- Tuberous sclerosis complex: 17% to 60% of these children have ASD, with a high likelihood of epilepsy as well[16]
- Fragile X: 30% to 50% show features of ASD
- 15q deletions: Angelman syndrome[17]
- Various metabolic conditions such as mitochondrial abnormalities, cerebral folate deficiency[18]
- Smith-Lemli-Opitz syndrome: 71% to 85% meet ASD criteria[19]
  - Autosomal Recessive disorder of cholesterol biosynthesis[15]

ROLE OF PRIMARY CARE PHYSICIAN

The primary care physician (PCP) most commonly initiates the workup for the diagnosis of ASD based on both parents' concerns and clinical suspicion from developmental milestone reviews at 18 to 24 months of age. The first diagnostic indicator of ASD that raises clinical suspicion for the PCP is often concern voiced by a parent. In addition to listening to the parent, the PCP can assess the child with a specific ASD screening tool (discussed in detail later). If the diagnosis of ASD is suspected, the PCP should proceed with a comprehensive medical assessment that includes a complete family and medical history, a detailed physical examination including a neurologic examination, and direct assessment of the child's social, language, and cognitive development.

Key outcomes of this comprehensive evaluation include[15,20,21]:

- Obtaining definitive diagnosis
- Excluding any differential diagnoses that may mimic ASD (**Box 1**)
- Identifying comorbid conditions that have implications for treatment or the need for genetic counseling
- Determining the child's level of functioning and profile of strengths and weaknesses

---

Box 1
Differential diagnosis of ASD

- Global developmental delay/intellectual disability
  - Social responsiveness and communication efforts are usually appropriate for developmental level
    - ASD: aberrant for their developmental level[15,21]
  - Usually can understand language at higher level than they can express
    - ASD: receptive language most affected[22]

- Pragmatic communication disorder
  - Persistent difficulties in the social use of verbal/nonverbal communication (inability to sustain conversation/unable to understand idioms/humor)
  - Absence of restricted repetitive patterns of behavior/interests/activities

- Developmental language disorder
  - Normal reciprocal social interactions, normal desire and intent to communicate, appropriate imaginative play[22]

- Hearing impairment
  - Normal reciprocal social interactions, imaginative play, normal eye-to-eye gaze, and facial expressions[15,22]

- Rett syndrome
  - Neurodevelopmental disorder almost exclusively in females
  - Loss of speech and purposeful hand movement at age 18 months

- Anxiety disorder/social phobia
  - Normal social and communication/language skills
  - ASD: inflexible to change in mannerisms/habits leading to anxiety/distress[22]

- Obsessive-compulsive disorder
  - Normal social and communication/language skills
  - Behavioral issues overlap with ASD[22]

- Language-based learning disability
  - Normal reciprocal social interactions, normal desire and intent to communicate, appropriate imaginative play
  - Difficulty or delay in processing content, but pragmatics intact

- Reactive attachment disorder
  - Similar to ASD; usually history of severe neglect or mental health issue in caretaker

Data from Refs.[15,21,22]

Ideally, once the PCP identifies a child at risk for ASD, he or she should initiate the referral process—utilizing a multidisciplinary approach to comprehensive evaluation to determine a definitive diagnosis of ASD. Each PCP has his or her own comfort level in dealing with children at risk for ASD. Once the PCP has completed a preliminary evaluation (at a minimum this evaluation should include documentation that the child's symptoms meet the DSM-5 or ICD-10 criteria),[2,3] a provisional diagnosis of ASD can be made. To prevent significant delay in treating the child while awaiting the definitive diagnosis, the PCP can simultaneously refer the child to start interventional therapy (ie, early intervention program if younger than 3 years, public school system if older than 3 years, speech therapy, occupational therapy, social worker, and audiologist).

There is no cure for ASD; however, early diagnosis and early intensive treatment have the potential to affect outcome in all aspects of ASD. According to a 2012 recommended guideline, treatment must be individualized depending on the specific behavioral and educational deficits of the child and the supportive needs of the family.[23]

To facilitate PCP competency in diagnosing ASD, the US Centers for Disease Control and Prevention, in collaboration with the American Academy of Pediatrics, initiated the Learn the Signs. Act Early campaign. This movement helped develop the autism ALARM initiative to promote improved surveillance and screening for ASD.[15]

- Autism is prevalent
- Listen to parents
  - Parents' concerns correlate with developmental problems in young children.[24]
- Act Early
  - An ASD-specific screening test should be performed anytime ASD concerns are raised during a developmental surveillance (**Box 2**).
  - The American Academy of Pediatrics recommends ASD screening at age 18 months and 24 months (grade 2C recommendation).[15]
- Refer
  - If results of ASD-specific screening are positive, refer for specialty evaluation and intervention without delay, even without definitive diagnosis.[15]
- Monitor
  - Continue to monitor every 6 to 12 months with long-term support is critical.[25]
  - Provide parents with information regarding parent groups, respite facilities, and other community-based support systems.
  - Provide parents with information regarding unconventional/unproven alternative therapies.[15,26,27]

Box 2
Surveillance of ASD

A child with ASD might:

- Not point at objects to show interest (point at airplane flying over)
- Not look at objects when another person points at them
- Have trouble relating to others; not have an interest in others
- Avoid eye contact and want to be alone
- Have trouble understanding other people's feelings or talking about their own feelings
- Prefer not to be held or cuddled or might cuddle when they want to
- Appear to be unaware when other people talk to them but respond to other sounds
- Be interested in people, but not know how to talk to, play with, or relate to them
- Repeat or echo words or phrases said to them; repeat words or phrases in place of normal language (echolalia)
- Have trouble expressing their needs using typical words/motions
- Not play pretend games (eg, pretend to feed a doll)
- Repeat actions over and over again
- Have trouble adapting when a routine changes
- Have unusual reactions to the way things smell, taste, look, feel, or sound
- Lose skills they once had (regression)

Data from Centers for Disease Control and Prevention. Autism Spectrum Disorder (ASD); Facts about ASD. Available at: www.cdc.gov/ncbddd/autism/facts.html. Accessed July 22, 2015.

     ○ Continue medical management for onset of seizures, sleep problems, nutritional issues, and behavioral/emotional difficulties.[26]

     ○ Monitor siblings for symptoms of ASD, language delay, learning difficulties, social problems, and anxiety/depression.[15,25]

COMPREHENSIVE EXAMINATION: PERSONAL/FAMILY HISTORY

A complete medical history should be obtained from the child's parents, teachers, and therapists for all children who screen positive for ASD.[3,28–30]

- Developmental history, with particular attention to early social-emotional and language milestones, play skills, behaviors, and any regression (important part of ASD spectrum; may be gradual or sudden)
- Hearing, vision, speech/language history and any parental concerns regarding each
- Specific information regarding early communicative behaviors, such as pointing, use of eye contact, and response to name
- History of repetitive, ritualized, or stereotyped behaviors, such as hand flapping
- Unusual visual behavior or preoccupation with parts of toys
- Frequent tantrums and trouble tolerating change or transition
- History of possible seizures
- Self-injury
- Significant disturbance in eating (pica) or sleep

Because ASD has a high genetic predisposition, a thorough 3-generation family history should be obtained. Specifically, parents should be questioned regarding the presence of the following disorders or concerns within the family[29,30]:

- ASD or any other previously termed diagnosis
- Language delay
- Intellectual disability
- Most common genetic disorders (as noted previously)
  - ○ Fragile X syndrome
  - ○ Angelman syndrome
  - ○ Prader-Willi syndrome
  - ○ Smith-Lemli-Opitz syndrome
  - ○ Tuberous sclerosis complex
- Learning and attentional disorders (eg, attention deficit disorder/attention deficit hyperactivity disorder)
- Anxiety/social phobia
- Obsessive-compulsive disorder
- Extreme shyness or mutism
- Mood disorders (depression)
- Schizophrenia
- Seizures
- Tic disorders
- Family dysfunction/stressors

PHYSICAL EXAMINATION

Adequate time should be allotted for evaluation of the child with suspected ASD, as communication/behavioral impairments may prove challenging. Important aspects of the examination should include[15,21]:

- Measurements of growth parameters; review of growth charts each office visit
  - Height and weight
    - ASD can cause dietary obsessions-compulsions or limitations owing to sensory issues resulting in nutritional concerns; body mass index should be assessed regularly.
  - Head circumference
    - Approximately one-fourth of ASD children have head circumference greater than the 97th percentile.[3,31]
    - Typically, acceleration of head growth occurs during the first year of life, followed by stabilization.
    - Head circumference may be related to abnormalities in early brain development in ASD children.
- Wood's lamp skin examination to rule out tuberous sclerosis
- Examination for dysmorphic features suggestive of an underlying genetic diagnosis or syndrome
- Muscle tone and reflexes
  - Check for hypotonia
  - Check for abnormal gait/clumsiness/toe walking
  - Address focal neurologic deficits or asymmetry through neuroimaging

ANCILLARY TESTING

Ancillary testing is a pertinent part of the comprehensive examination for exclusion of mimicking conditions, for inclusion of potentially treatable associated conditions of ASD, and for definition of child's strengths and weaknesses to aid in education planning. Ancillary examinations should include[21,25,32]:

- Vision and hearing assessments
- Speech, language, and communication assessments
- Developmental/intelligence testing with separate estimates for verbal and nonverbal skills
- Assessment of adaptive skills to document the presence or absence of associated intellectual disability
- Neuropsychological or achievement testing
- Sensorimotor or occupational therapy evaluation

ADDITIONAL EVALUATION

Once a child has a positive ASD screening or a confirmed ASD diagnosis, further evaluation may be warranted to help exclude certain differential diagnoses and to identify any comorbidities that may have important implications for treatment.[25] Additionally, further testing may aid in establishing the etiology of the child's ASD, which can provide emotional relief to the parents and serve as an important prognosticator of the disorder. The PCP/ASD specialist may organize supplementary laboratory testing, as indicated, to rule out lead poisoning (if pica is present) and disorders of amino acids, carbohydrate, purine, peptide, and mitochondrial metabolism as plausible etiologies.[25,33,34] Routine use of the aforementioned metabolic testing, along with any neuroimaging examination, which would include an MRI or electroencephalography, is not indicated, and in the absence of clinical signs or symptoms produces a low yield in diagnosing ASD.[33]

Genetic counseling should be offered with confirmed diagnosis of ASD.[10] This counseling should include chromosomal microarray and DNA analysis for fragile

X syndrome.[18] Any other specific genetic testing should be guided by the child's individual clinical profile. The reason for genetic counseling is the increased risk of ASD in siblings of children with a genetic cause of the ASD, which may affect the decision for future pregnancies (standard prevalence of a sibling having ASD for an isolated etiology of the disorder is 4%–7%).[18]

SURVEILLANCE/SCREENING: EARLY INDICATORS

A 2006 systematic review using family home videos found that children can show signs and symptoms of ASD as early as 6 months of age. The review continued to document that during the first year of life, the behaviors that were most consistently altered in ASD children were reduced frequency of looking at faces and reduced response to name. During year 2 of life, sharing experiences, interests, or attention with others were the most common modified behaviors.[35] As noted earlier, most signs and symptoms are measurable by 18 to 24 months of age and remain stable through the duration of toddlerhood to preschool to school age[25] (**Box 3**).

OTHER RED FLAGS

Other important early symptoms and signs of ASD include, but are not limited to[15,25]:

- Parental concerns about deficits in social skills
- Parental concerns about deficits in language skills or behavior
- Parental concerns about frequent tantrums or intolerance to change
- Delayed language and social or communication skills
- No single words by 16 months
- Lack of pretend or symbolic play by 18 months

Box 3
Early signs of autism

Gaze

- Lack of appropriate gaze
- Lack of warm, joyful expressions with gaze

Receptive language

- Lack of recognition of mother's/father's voice
- Lack of response to name by 12 months of age
- Increased awareness of environmental sounds
- Lack of interest in or response to comments made by others

Expressive language

- Lack of to-and-fro pattern of vocalization that typically occurs by 6 months of age
- No babbling before 9 months of age
- Lack of expressions such as "uh-oh" and "huh"

Prespeech gestures

- Decrease or absent use of prespeech gestures, such as waving/pointing/showing by 12 months of age

Data from Johnson CP, Myers SM. Identification and evaluation of children with autism spectrum disorders. Pediatrics 2007;120:1183.

- No spontaneous, meaningful (not repetitive or echolalic) 2-word phrases by 24 months
- Loss or regression of any language or social skills at any age

SURVEILLANCE/SCREENING: FORMAL TOOLS

The American Academy of Pediatrics and the American Academy of Neurology recommend screening of all pediatric patients and early diagnosis in the evaluation and management of children with ASD.[15,25] In contrast, the US Preventive Service Task Force and the American Academy of Family Physician (AAFP) recommend screening in only symptomatic pediatric populations (the US Preventive Service Task Force released a Draft Recommendation Statement on August 31, 2015 stating Insufficient Evidence in screening all pediatric patients for ASD).[36] PCPs should use ASD-specific screening tools to augment general developmental screening tools. ASD-specific tools systematically address items specific to the core symptoms of ASD. These precise screening tools should be used in the following children[15,25,37]:

- Children with delayed language or communication milestones
- Children who have a regression in social or language skills
- Children who have siblings with ASD
- All children at 18 and 24 months of age (grade 2C recommendation)
- Children, regardless of age, whose parents, care provider, or clinician raise concerns regarding ASD

It is recommended that any child with a positive ASD-specific screen be referred for developmental services as soon as possible (grade 1B recommendation).[15,30]

ASD screening tools are categorized into 2 tiers. The first-tier screen is the basic ASD-specific tool that is used to identify children at risk for ASD and is the tool of choice for first-time screeners. In comparison, the longer, more time consuming second-tier screen is used to discriminate ASD from other developmental disorders in children that have had a positive first-tier screen. One limitation of the current ASD-specific screens is that they have limited sensitivity and specificity because of the complex continuum of ASD. For optimal utilization, a first-tier screen should be more sensitive than specific.[30] Keep in mind that the age of the child and severity of symptoms affect the sensitivity and specificity of each test. A brief overview of the more frequently used screening tools follows:

- Checklist for Autism in Toddlers
  - Age: 18 to 24 months
  - Basis: parent report/observation report
  - 20% sensitivity; 98% specificity
  - Second-tier
- Modified Checklist for Autism in Toddlers
  - Age 16 to 30 months
  - Basis: 20-point questionnaire by parent
  - 85% sensitivity; 98% specificity
  - First-tier screen
- Screening Tool for Autism in Two-Year-Olds
  - Age: 24 to 36 months
  - Basis: 12 observed activities/20-minute play session; requires specific training
  - 92% to 95% sensitive
- Infant Toddler Checklist
  - Age: 6 to 24 months
  - Basis: 24-point questionnaire by parent

- Social Communication Questionnaire
  - Age: 4 to 40 years
  - Basis: 40-point questionnaire by parent
  - Sensitivity 85%; specificity 75%
  - Not a first tier
- Childhood Autism Syndrome Test
  - Age: 4 to 11 years
  - Basis: 37-point questionnaire by parent
  - Sensitivity/specificity varies
  - Not a first tier
- Autism Spectrum Screening Questionnaire
  - Age: 7 to 16 years
  - Basis: 27-point questionnaire by both parent and teacher
  - Sensitivity/specificity varies
  - First-tier for high-functioning ASD
- Autism Spectrum Quotient–Children's Version
  - Age 4 to 11 years
  - Basis: parent report
  - Sensitivity 95%; specificity 95%

MANAGEMENT GOALS

The overall basis for management of ASD is 3-fold: (1) maximize function, (2) promote the child's independence, (3) improve quality of life (**Fig. 1**).[23] To accomplish these 3 goals, a comprehensive, individualized treatment approach is required. Although there is no cure for ASD, early diagnosis and intervention are the foundation for optimal outcomes. Using a multidisciplinary methodology based on the child's and family's strengths and weakness, symptoms can be optimized.[38] This multidisciplinary approach may include the following providers[39]:

- PCP
- Developmental pediatrician, child neurologist, child psychiatrist
- Psychologist or neuropsychologist

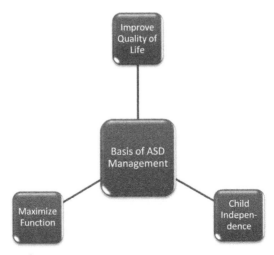

Fig. 1. Management of ASD.

- Geneticist or genetics counselor
- Speech language pathologist
- Occupational therapist
- Audiologist
- Social worker

Early intervention programs (provided by most states for kids before entry into pre-school), school-based education programs (via the use of an individualized education plan), or private practice therapists are a few of the avenues of treatment that children with ASD and their families can access.

In the United States, the Individuals with Disabilities Education Act guarantees a free and appropriate public education for every child with a disability, including children with ASD.[40] Each state is responsible for implementing and enforcing its own Individuals with Disabilities Education Act policies. Insurance coverage is also available in most states for ASD treatment.

The role of the PCP in the medical management of ASD is plentiful. Not only does the PCP most likely initiate the early identification of ASD, the PCP may provide a patient-centered medical home for children with ASD.[39] This approach entails provision of routine health maintenance including anticipatory guidance, preventive care, and care coordination and support, guidance, and advocacy for family members.

The PCP can provide surveillance for several comorbidities that children with ASD may develop. These may include[41]:

- Medical disorders (seizures; lead poisoning from pica)
- Developmental and mental health comorbidities (hyperactivity, anxiety/depression)
- Sleep problems (late onset, frequent sleep walking), which might affect daytime functioning
- Gastrointestinal, feeding, and nutrition problems (constipation, calcium/vitamin D deficiency)
- Delays in acquisition of self-help skills (toileting, dressing, hygiene)

As far as support, guidance, and advocacy for families, the PCP plays a critical role. The PCP can help the family understand the essential components of the treatment program and which types of programs have evidence of benefit, including the potential benefits and risks of complementary and alternative therapies. PCPs should be aware of which local or national organizations provide autism intervention or support in their communities so that they can guide families appropriately.[42]

PHARMACOLOGIC STRATEGIES

Psychopharmacologic agents do not treat the core deficits of ASD; however, they can improve the child's functioning and the ability to participate in behavioral therapy. Psychopharmacologic medications should be initiated only when educational and behavioral interventions are in place and maximized. If medications are prescribed, physicians need to monitor closely for adverse side effects and start at lower doses and with slower titrations, as ASD children are more sensitive to psychopharmacotherapy than non-ASD children.[43] PCPs who undertake the prescription writing of psychotropic agents may need to do so in consultation with a health professional with particular expertise in ASD.

Inattention and Hyperactivity

Inattention, hyperactivity, and disorganized symptoms in ASD may be related to comorbid attention deficit hyperactivity disorder or to other factors that affect function such as overarousal or anxiety.[44] Recommended medication, for both inattention and hyperactivity, is methylphenidate (grade 2A recommendation). Risperidone and dextroamphetamine are also beneficial for hyperactivity.

Maladaptive Behaviors

Symptoms of maladaptive behavior include irritability, aggression, explosive outbursts, and self-injury. Recommended medication is risperidone (Grade 2A recommendation).[45] However, these behaviors may occur in response to anxiety, mood disorders, or impulse control issues; if so, then medication to target the particular condition is the best option.[43]

Repetitive Behaviors

Repetitive behaviors, similar to the mannerisms seen in obsessive compulsive disorder, often interfere with daily functioning in adults with ASD. Recommended medication in adults is fluoxetine (Prozac) (grade 2C recommendation)[46]; however, a 2013 Cochrane review found no evidence to support fluoxetine or selective serotonin reuptake inhibitors (SSRIs) in general, in children with ASD for these repetitive behaviors alone.[47]

Anxiety

Anxiety is common in individuals with ASD and may contribute to aggressive, explosive, or self-injurious behaviors. Recommended medication for anxiety is any SSRI (grade 2B recommendation).[48]

Dysregulated Mood

Recommended medication is an atypical antipsychotic or SSRI (grade 2C recommendation).

Depressive Mood

Recommended medication in adults is an SSRI (grade 2B recommendation).[47]

Other Conditions

Seizures are more common in children with ASD than the general population. Pharmacologic management of seizures in children with ASD is similar to that of non-ASD children.

Gastrointestinal problems seen in ASD children are constipation, gastroesophageal reflux disease, chronic abdominal pain, and chronic diarrhea. A 2010 systematic review found a lack of high-quality data regarding pharmacotherapy for these symptoms in children with ASD in particular; therefore, recommendations are no change between non-ASD and ASD treatment.[49]

Sleep disturbance may be related to abnormalities in melatonin, serotonin, or γ-amino butyric acid. No medication is approved by the US Food and Drug Administration for use in sleep in ASD. In a 2011 meta-analysis, melatonin, doses ranging from 1 to 10 mg, may be effective in helping children with ASD to fall asleep and sleep longer when taken 30 minutes before bedtime.[50]

NONPHARMACOLOGIC STRATEGIES

Intensive behavioral and educational interventions are the primary component of treatment programs for ASD.[26] Despite the lack of evidence from randomized, controlled trials owing to practical and ethical factors, there is growing evidence from observational studies and systemic reviews that children with ASD should participate in therapeutic programs as early as possible.[23,26,51] The National Research Council recommends that educational services include a minimum of 25 hours a week, 12 months per year, in which the child is engaged in systematically planned and developmentally appropriate educational activity toward identified objectives.[51] Most research has been centered on preschool and school-age children with little evidence about treatment of ASD in adolescents or children younger than 2 years.[30]

Children with ASD generally require a combination of therapies and interventions to address their individual constellation of symptoms. A systematic review found insufficient evidence to suggest that any particular interventional model was superior over another one.[23] Three broad conceptual models are categorized as follows (with a combined fourth model):

1. Intensive behavioral intervention model
   a. Based on principles of behavioral modification
   b. Targets the core of ASD
   c. Example: applied behavior analysis
   d. Systematic reviews of randomized, controlled trials = established treatment option
2. Structured teaching model
   a. Helps ASD individuals overcome areas of weakness
   b. Individualized to student; includes family involvement
   c. 2011 systematic review = some evidence of benefit in cognitive and motor function[52]
3. Developmental/relationship model
   a. Focused on teaching skills that are essential to development
   b. Current evidence = inconclusive
4. Integrative model
   a. Combines more than one interventional model

Other behavioral/educational models available to children with ASD include communication intervention (insufficient evidence to support a specific methodology for improvement of communication skills), sensory integration therapy (controversial and evidence regarding its benefit is inconsistent), and occupational therapy (little research regarding traditional occupational therapy).

COMPLEMENTARY AND ALTERNATIVE MEDICINE

Complementary and alternative medicine therapies have been used to help treat the core symptoms of ASD: inattention, sleep disturbance, gastrointestinal and symptoms and to promote overall good health.[53] Despite the lack of high-quality evidence, some families still are interested in trying complementary and alternative medicine. The PCP should be open to discuss such options and provide guidance of known safety issues or harmful side effects.

SUMMARY

ASD is a complex disorder that is becoming more prevalent. Because of this increased prevalence, PCPs must become more knowledgeable about ASD so they can provide appropriate screening, evaluation, and treatment as part of an interdisciplinary team and to serve patients and families within the medical home.

REFERENCES

1. Developmental Disabilities Monitoring Network Surveillance Year 2010 Principal Investigators, Centers for Disease Control and Prevention (CDC). Prevalence of autism spectrum disorder among children aged 8 years – autism and developmental disabilities monitoring network, 11 sites, United States, 2010. MMWR Surveill Summ 2014;63(2):1–21.
2. American Psychiatric Association. Autism spectrum disorder. In: Diagnostic and statistical manual of mental disorders. 5th edition. Arlington (VA): American Psychiatric Association; 2013. p. 50.
3. World Health Organization. The ICD-10 Classification of Mental and Behavioural Disorders. Clinical descriptions and diagnostic guidelines. Available at: http://www.who.int/classifications/icd/en/bluebook.pdf. Accessed July 30, 2015.
4. Fombonne E. Epidemiology of pervasive developmental disorders. Pediatr Res 2009;65:591.
5. Chawarksa K, Klin A, Paul R, et al. Autism spectrum disorder in the second year: stability and change in syndrome expression. J Child Psychol Psychiatry 2007; 48:128.
6. Wiggins LD, Baio J, Rice C. Examination of the time between first evaluation and first autism spectrum diagnosis in a population-based sample. J Dev Behav Pediatr 2006;27:S79.
7. Howlin P, Moorf A. Diagnosis in autism: a survey of over 1200 patients in the UK. Autism 1997;1:135.
8. Constantino JN, Zhang Y, Frazier T, et al. Sibling recurrence and the genetic epidemiology of autism. Am J Psychiatry 2010;167:1349.
9. Sandin S, Lichtenstein P, Kuja-Halkola R, et al. The familial risk of autism. JAMA 2014;311:1770.
10. Muhle R, Trentacoste SV, Rapin I. The genetics of autism. Pediatrics 2004;113: e472.
11. Reichenberg A, Gross R, Weiser M, et al. Advancing paternal age and autism. Arch Gen Psychiatry 2006;63:1026.
12. Sandin S, Hultman CM, Kolevzon A, et al. Advancing maternal age is associated with increasing risk for autism: a review and meta-analysis. J Am Acad Child Adolesc Psychiatry 2012;51:477.
13. Jain A, Marshall J, Bikema A, et al. Autism occurrence by MMR vaccine status among US children with older siblings with and without autism. JAMA 2015; 313(15):1534–40.
14. Bertrand J, Mars A, Boyle C, et al. Prevalence of autism in a United States population: the Brick Towship, New Jersey, investigation. Pediatrics 2001;108:1155.
15. Johnson CP, Myers SM, American Academy of Pediatrics Council on Children with Disabilities. Identification and evaluation of children with autism spectrum disorders. Pediatrics 2007;120:1183.
16. Smalley SL. Autism and tuberous sclerosis. J Autism Dev Disord 1998;28:407.
17. Veltman MW, Craig EE, Bolton PF. Autism spectrum disorders in Prader-Willi and Angleman syndromes: a systemic review. Psychiatr Genet 2005;15:243.
18. Schaefer GB, Mendelsohn NJ, Professional Practice and Guidelines Committee. Clinical genetics evaluation in identifying the etiology of autism spectrum disorders: 2013 guideline revisions. Genet Med 2013;15:399.
19. Sikora DM, Pettit-Kekel K, Penfield J, et al. The near universal presence of autism spectrum disorders in children with Smith-Lemli-Opitz syndrome. Am J Med Genet A 1511;2006:140.

20. Filipek PA, Accardo PJ, Baranek GT, et al. The screening and diagnosis of autistic spectrum disorders. J Autism Dev Disord 1999;29:439.
21. Volkmar F, Siegel M, Woodbury-Smith M, et al. Practice parameter for the assessment and treatment of children and adolescents with autism spectrum disorder. J Am Acad Child Adolesc Psychiatry 2014;53:237.
22. Teplin SW. Autism and related disorders. In: Levine MD, Carey WB, Crocker AC, editors. Developmental behavioral pediatrics. 3rd edition. Philadelphia: WB Saunders; 1999. p. 589.
23. Maglione MA, Gans D, Das L, et al. Nonmedical interventions for children with ASD: recommended guidelines and further research needs. Pediatrics 2012; 130(Suppl 2):S169.
24. Glascoe FP, Dworkin PH. The role of parents in the detection of developmental and behavioral problems. Pediatrics 1995;95:829.
25. Filipek PA, Accardo PJ, Ashwal S, et al. Practice parameter: screening and diagnosis of autism: report of the Quality Standards Subcommittee of the American Academy of neurology and the Child Neurology Society. Neurology 2000;55:468.
26. Myers SM, Johnson CP, American Academy of Pediatrics Council on Children with Disabilities. Management of children with autism spectrum disorders. Pediatrics 2007;120:1162.
27. Rapin I. Autism. N Engl J Med 1997;337:97.
28. Dworkin PH. Detection of behavioral, developmental, and psychosocial problems in pediatric primary care practice. Curr Opin Pediatr 1993;5:531.
29. Howlin P, Asgharian A. The diagnosis of autism and Asperger syndrome: findings from a survey of 770 families. Dev Med Child Neurol 1999;41:834.
30. Zwaigenbaum L, Bryson S, Lord C, et al. Clinical assessment and management of toddlers with suspected autism spectrum disorder: insights from studies of high-risk infants. Pediatrics 2009;123:1383.
31. Lainhart JE, Piven J, Wzorek M, et al. Macrocephaly in children and adults with autism. J Am Acad Child Adolesc Psychiatry 1997;36:282.
32. Dover CJ, Le Couteur A. How to diagnose autism. Arch Dis Child 2007;92:540.
33. Battaglia A, Carey JC. Etiologic yield of autistic spectrum disorders: a prospective study. Am J Med Genet C Semin Med Genet 2006;142C:3.
34. Manzi B, Loizzo AL, Giana G, et al. Autism and metabolic diseases. J Child Neurol 2008;23:307.
35. Paloma R, Belin chon M, Ozonoff S. Autism and family home videos: a comprehensive review. J Dev Behav Pediatr 2006;27:S59.
36. Draft Update Summary: Autism Spectrum Disorder in Young Children: Screening. U.S. Preventive Services Task Force. Available at: http://www.uspreventiveservicestaskforce.org/Page/Document/UpdateSummaryDraft/autism-spectrum-disorder-in-young-children-screening. Accessed July 22, 2015.
37. Council on Children with Disabilities, Section on Developmental Behavioral Pediatrics, Bright Futures Steering Committee, Medical Home Initiatives for Children with Special Needs Project Advisory Committee. Identifying infants and young children with developmental disorders in the medical home: an algorithm for developmental surveillance and screening. Pediatrics 2006;118:405.
38. Orinstein AJ, Helt M, Troy E, et al. Intervention for optimal outcome in children and adolescents with a history of autism. J Dev Behav Pediatr 2014;35:247.
39. Carbone PS, Farley M, Davis T. Primary care for children with autism. Am Fam Physician 2010;81:453.

40. Public Law 108-446. Individuals with Disabilities Education Improvement Act of 2004. Available at: www.copyright.gov/legistlation/pl108-446.pdf. Accessed May 20, 2010.

41. Brimacombe M, Chaaban J, Zimmerman-Bier B, et al. Autism spectrum disorders: concurrent clinical disorders. J Child Neurol 2008;23:6.

42. Committee on Children with Disabilities. American Academy of Pediatrics: the pediatrician's role in the diagnosis and management of autistic spectrum disorder in children. Pediatrics 2001;107:1221.

43. Towbin KE. Strategies for pharmacological treatment of high functioning autism and Asperger syndrome. Child Adolesc Psychiatr Clin N Am 2003;12:23.

44. Huffman LC, Sutcliffe TL, Tanner IS, et al. Management of symptoms in children with autism spectrum disorders: a comprehensive review of pharmacologic and complementary-alternative medicine treatments. J Dev Behav Pediatr 2011;32:56.

45. Shea S, Turgay A, Carroll A, et al. Risperidone in the treatment of disruptive behavioral symptoms in children with autistic and other pervasive developmental disorders. Pediatrics 2004;114:e634.

46. Carrasco M, Volkmar FR, Block MH. Pharmacologic treatment of repetitive behaviors in autism spectrum disorders: evidence of publication bias. Pediatrics 2012; 129:e1301.

47. Williams K, Brignell A, Randall M, et al. Selective serotonin reuptake inhibitors (SSRIs) for autism spectrum disorders (ASD). Cochrane Database Syst Rev 2013;(8):CD004677.

48. Ipser JC, Stein DJ, Hawkridge S, et al. Pharmacotherapy for anxiety disorders in children and adolescents. Cochrane Database Syst Rev 2009;(8):CD005170.

49. Buie T, Fuchs GJ 3rd, Furuta GT, et al. Recommendations for evaluation and treatment of common gastrointestinal problems in children with ASDs. Pediatrics 2010;125(Suppl 1):S1.

50. Rossignol DA, Frye RE. Melatonin in autism spectrum disorders: a systematic review and meta-analysis. Dev Med Child Neurol 2011;53:783.

51. National Research Council. Committee on Educational Interventions for children with Autism. In: Lord C, McGee JP, editors. Educating children with autism. Washington, DC: National Academy Press; 2001. p. 150–4.

52. Warren Z, Veenstra-VanderWeele J, Stone W, et al. Therapies for children with autism spectrum disorders. AHRQ Publication No.11-EHC029-EF. Rockville (MD): Agency for Healthcare Research and Quality; 2011. p. 106.

53. Hanson E, La Kalish, Bunce E, et al. Use of complementary and alternative medicine among children diagnosed with autism spectrum disorder. J Autism Dev Disord 2007;37:628.

Eating Disorders in the Primary Care Setting

Devdutta Sangvai, MD, MBA

KEYWORDS

• Eating disorder • Anorexia nervosa • Bulimia nervosa • Binge eating disorder

KEY POINTS

- Primary care providers, in conjunction with therapists and nutritionists, can provide treatment for patients with less complex eating disorders.
- Eating disorders more commonly are diagnosed in white adolescent girls or young women, but other ethnic groups and men are also at risk, particularly with binge eating disorder.
- A primary goal in the treatment of all eating disorders is restoration to ideal body weight.
- In the absence of psychiatric comorbidities, there are few approved medications for eating disorders.

Eating disorders (ED), a complex set of illnesses, most commonly affect adolescent girls and young women.[1,2] Because primary care providers (PCPs) are likely to be the first, and sometimes only, physicians who encounter these patients, it is important for them to be able to diagnose and treat, or refer. Early diagnosis and treatment are associated with a higher rate of recovery, and extended illness is associated with potentially devastating consequences. At the same time, not all adolescent girls, young women, and men who are preoccupied with weight and body image present with ED. Careful attention to signs and symptoms, along with a welcoming, safe environment that allows for honest dialogue, will enable the physician to identify and treat patients with ED. Treatment commonly involves a team-based approach in which the PCP plays an integral role, along with a therapist and nutritionist. More complex patients may require the expertise of a psychiatrist and other medical specialists. For the less complex patient, the PCP can lend a whole-body approach to care, including the diagnosis and treatment of comorbid psychiatric conditions, such as depression and anxiety.

This article focuses on outpatient diagnosis and management of ED in adolescent and adult populations. Diagnosis and treatment of children, particularly premenarchal girls, largely follow the guidance set for adolescents and adults; however, additional attention needs to be placed on metabolic disorders, developmental considerations, growth rate, and other early milestones in the pediatric population.[3]

The author has nothing to disclose.
Department of Community and Family Medicine, Duke University School of Medicine, 718 Rutherford Street, Durham, NC 27705, USA
E-mail address: devdutta.sangvai@duke.edu

Prim Care Clin Office Pract 43 (2016) 301–312
http://dx.doi.org/10.1016/j.pop.2016.01.007
0095-4543/16/$ – see front matter © 2016 Elsevier Inc. All rights reserved.

DIAGNOSTIC AND STATISTICAL MANUAL OF MENTAL DISORDERS, 5TH EDITION, AND EATING DISORDERS

Although ED are perceived to be a very recent phenomena, accelerated by cultural norms that emphasize thinness, anorexia nervosa (AN) was listed in the first Diagnostic and Statistical Manual of Mental Disorders (DSM-1) in 1952.[4] Indeed, descriptions of AN occur throughout history. The numbers of these illnesses have, however, increased over time.[5] This increase is likely related to cultural expectations and improved awareness among health care providers. It should be noted, however, that the relatively poor prognosis of AN did not change over the 20th century.[6] Binge eating disorder (BED) was included in DSM-5, published in 2013.

DSM-5 categorizes disorders of feeding and eating into 7 main groups. This article focuses on the 3 (**Table 1**) that are most likely to present in the PCP environment:

- AN
  ○ Restrictive subtype
  ○ Binge-purge subtype (AN-BP)
- Bulimia nervosa (BN)
- BED

Although DSM-5 provides explicit criteria and terminology to help aid in classification and establishment of a diagnosis, it is important to remember that patients with ED may not meet all criteria, and presentation may therefore be mixed and variable over time. Moreover, in the initial stage of illness, a patient may present to the PCP with more traditional primary care and/or somatic complaints that could represent an early signal that an ED workup is warranted. It is important to remember that early diagnosis and treatment may to lead to improved outcomes.[7,8] Fortunately, treatment approaches to subclinical cases largely mirror that for more definitive instances. From a practical standpoint, intervening when weight loss is less and behaviors are less entrenched and medical complications less severe may prove easier than when signs and symptoms are more pronounced.

Fear of weight gain and Criterion B for anorexia must also be applied in the context of dieting, social norms, and other factors leading to weight dissatisfaction.[9] Not all fear of gaining weight is a positive finding suggestive of Criterion B. Similarly, although individuals with ED may focus on a particular area of the body with which they are dissatisfied (commonly the abdomen, hips, and buttocks), preoccupation, repetitive behaviors, and impairment in social functioning related to this dissatisfaction are more consistent with body dysmorphic disorder than an ED.[10]

Patients rarely present to the PCP with a chief complaint of "eating disorder"; more commonly, patients present with one or more primary care complaints that signal signs or symptoms of ED behavior, including fatigue, cold intolerance, menstrual irregularity, or gastrointestinal (GI) issues such as abdominal pain and constipation.[11] Others may present with changes in weight as a chief complaint. Some patients, particularly those who visit the office with a parent, may present with a direct concern about an ED. Older patients may reluctantly present at the urging of a friend or loved one, stating something similar to, "my friend thinks I have an issue with my eating," or "my boyfriend caught me purging". Because most patients do not present with a complaint of ED, the suspicion will likely emerge during an interview for a more traditional primary care issue during which the patient is asked about appetite and food intake. **Box 1** lists common responses to questions about food intake that warrant formal screening.

Table 1
Diagnostic criteria for anorexia nervosa, bulimia nervosa, and binge eating disorder

AN	A. Restriction of energy intake relative to requirements, leading to a significantly low body weight in the context of age, sex, developmental trajectory, and physical health. Significantly low weight is defined as a weight that is less than minimally normal or, for children and adolescents, less than that minimally expected.	ICD-9-CM 307.1
	B. Intense fear of gaining weight or of becoming fat, or persistent behavior that interferes with weight gain, even though at a significantly low weight.	
	C. Disturbance in the way in which one's body weight or shape is experienced, undue influence of body weight or shape on self-evaluation, or persistent lack of recognition of the seriousness of the current low body weight.	
BN	A. Recurrent episodes of binge eating. An episode of binge eating is characterized by both of the following: 1. Eating, in a discrete period of time (eg, within any 2-h period) an amount of food that is definitely larger than what most individuals would eat in a similar period of time under similar circumstances. 2. A sense of lack of control over eating during the episode (eg, a feeling that one cannot stop eating or control what or how much one is eating).	307.51 (F50.2)
	B. Recurrent inappropriate compensatory behaviors in order to prevent weight gain, such as self-induced vomiting; misuse of laxatives, diuretics, or other medications; fasting; or excessive exercise.	
	C. The binge eating and inappropriate compensatory behaviors both occur, on average, at least once a week for 3 mo.	
	D. Self-evaluation is unduly influenced by body shape and weight.	
	E. The disturbance does not occur exclusively during episodes of AN.	
BED	A. Recurrent episodes of binge eating. An episode of binge eating is characterized by both of the following: 1. Eating, in a discrete period of time (eg, within any 2-h period) an amount of food that is definitely larger than what most people would eat in a similar period of time under similar circumstances. 2. A sense of lack of control over eating during the episode (eg, a feeling that one cannot stop eating or control what or how much one is eating).	307.51 (F50.8)
	B. The binge-eating episodes are associated with 3 (or more) of the following: 1. Eating much more rapidly than normal. 2. Eating until feeling uncomfortably full. 3. Eating large amounts of food when not feeling physically hungry. 4. Eating alone because of feeling embarrassed by how much one is eating. 5. Feeling disgusted with oneself, depressed, or very guilty afterward.	
	C. Marked distress regarding binge eating is present.	
	D. The binge eating is not associated with the recurrent use of inappropriate compensatory behavior as in BN and does not occur exclusively during the course of BN or AN.	

Box 1
Red flag responses to questions about appetite and food intake

I am just not hungry and don't feel comfortable forcing myself to eat.

I am too busy and sometimes forget to eat.

I cannot find foods that I like to eat. (This statement coupled with a recent change in diet that limits food warrants additional questioning.)

Whenever I eat something, I feel sick.

SCREENING FOR EATING DISORDERS

There are several tools that can be used to screen for ED, some that are in-depth and multiquestion and more suitable for the mental health setting. Given the time demands in the PCP setting, a short tool, such as the SCOFF or Eating Disorder Screen for Primary Care (ESP) questionnaire, is more practical (**Table 2**).

Given its low sensitivity of 53.7% (specificity of 93.5%),[12] PCPs should supplement the SCOFF with questions about family history of ED, affective disorders, or activities that promote thinness (eg, some athletics, modeling). The ESP is a similar short 5-question screening instrument used to detect ED. Answering no to question 1 or yes to the other 4 questions indicates an abnormal response. Two or more abnormal responses to the questions indicate a positive screen result. Here too, a positive screen must be supplemented with additional questions to enable a provisional or definitive diagnosis vis-à-vis DSM-5 criteria.

Table 2
SCOFF and eating disorder screen for primary care for screening for eating disorder

SCOFF	ESP
Do you make yourself *Sick* because you feel uncomfortably full?	Are you satisfied with your eating patterns?
Do you worry you have lost *Control* over how much you eat?	Have any members of your family suffered with an eating disorder?
Have you recently lost more than *One* stone (7.7 kg) in a 3-mo period?	Do you ever eat in secret?
Do you believe yourself to be *Fat* when others say you are too thin?	Does your weight affect the way you feel about yourself?
Would you say that *Food* dominates your life?	Do you currently suffer with or have you ever suffered in the past with an eating disorder?
SCORE: One point is given for every "yes" answer. A score of ≥ 2 indicates a concern for ED.	*SCORE:* "No" to the first question or "yes" to the other 4 questions indicates an abnormal response.

From Cotton MA, Ball C, Robinson P. Four simple questions can help screen for eating disorders. J Gen Intern Med 2003;18(1):53–4; with permission.

ANOREXIA NERVOSA

Among the more physically recognizable (because of potential for emaciated appearance) and serious ED, AN is marked by significantly decreased net caloric intake, fear of weight gain, and body-image disturbance, commonly without the ability to recognize the seriousness of health status. Patients with AN can be very rational about cause and effect with other aspects of their own health and the health of others, but cannot make the same connection with their disordered eating. The prevalence of AN is 0.3% to 1.0% among women[13] (assuming a panel size of 2500 patients for a full-time family physician, the average physician could have as many as 38–125 female patients with AN). Less is known about the prevalence in men; however, some have placed the prevalence of ED in men at 10% to 15% of the ED population. Although AN occurs across industrialized nations, it is less common among Latino, Asian, and African American than white populations. By some estimates, the prevalence is increasing among non-white individuals.[14]

Because of the age at onset and the severe restriction in nutrition, AN can lead to serious long-term developmental consequences, including failure to meet expected growth and low bone mineral density.[15] The physical presentations of AN can be ascribed to starvation. Common findings include amenorrhea or delay in menarche, hypotension, hypothermia, and bradycardia.[16] Laboratory test results may indicate anemia, leukopenia, elevated urea nitrogen, elevated hepatic enzymes, and endocrine abnormalities.[16] As such, an initial workup should include a complete blood count with white blood cell differential, complete metabolic profile, and thyroid laboratory tests. A baseline electrocardiogram may also provide additional insight into patients presenting with hypotension and/or bradycardia. Bone densitometry should also be considered, particularly for the individual who has been severely underweight for an extended period of time.[17] **Table 3** lists the medical complications of ED and can serve as a guide in individualizing the patient's workup.

Many AN patients will have normal laboratory test and other results and no physical findings on examination, other than low weight or failure to meet expected developmental goals. Management of any laboratory test result abnormalities must include consideration of whether the abnormality is primary or secondary to ED. For example, hypokalemia in a patient with AN (binge/purge subtype) will usually resolve over time as purging ceases, and there may be no need for exogenous potassium supplementation. For many patients with AN, an exhaustive diagnostic workup will show few to no clinical abnormalities. It can prove challenging to the PCP aiming to convince a patient who may be reticent to accept an ED diagnosis. Furthermore, it may inadvertently validate to the patient that her current patterns of eating, exercise, and other are not harmful. To avoid these pitfalls, the PCP should inform the patient that laboratory results and tests help support making the diagnosis but are not the only issues to consider.

Severity of AN is characterized by body mass index (BMI) as outlined in **Table 4**. There are 2 subtypes of AN, restricting type and binge-eating/purging type. As the names imply, the restricting type does not typically engage in binge eating or purging behaviors, whereas the binge-eating/purging type indicates recurrent episodes of bingeing-purging.

Although most purging in AN-BP (as well as in BN discussed later) involves self-induced vomiting, other forms of activity and other behaviors can have the same net effect. As such, the PCP suspecting an eating disorder should inquire about not only purging in the form of vomiting but also other purgatives, including laxatives, diuretics, and excessive exercise. When any of these are present, the history interview and workup should be refined. For example, a patient with AN who is over-exercising may have musculoskeletal symptoms that are better explained by overuse and dehydration than electrolytic abnormalities.

A primary goal of ED treatment is weight restoration to ideal body weight (IBW). There is considerable debate on how to calculate IBW,[18] and the PCP needs to factor

Table 3 Medical complications of eating disorders			
Organ System	AN[16]	BN[16]	BED
Cardiovascular	Bradycardia and hypotension Mitral valve prolapse Sudden death (related to QT prolongation) Peripheral edema Refeeding syndrome	Arrhythmias Diet pill toxicity: palpitations, hypertension Emitine cardiomyopathy Mitral valve prolapse	Hypertension secondary to obesity Hyperlipidemia secondary to diet and obesity
Dermatologic	Dry skin Carotenodermia Lanugo hair Starvation-associated pruritis	—	Diabetic skin changes Skin changes due to morbid obesity
GI	Constipation Refeeding pancreatitis Acute gastric dilatation due to refeeding	Dental erosion Parotid gland swelling Esophageal rupture Gastroesophageal reflux due to chronic relaxation of the sphincter Acute gastric dilatation After-binge pancreatitis Constipation due to laxative abuse Cathartic colon	Bloating Abdominal pain
Endocrine and metabolic	Amenorrhea Infertility Osteoporosis Thyroid abnormalities Hypercortisolemia Hypercholesterolemia due to impaired cholesterol metabolism Hypoglycemia Neurogenic diabetes insipidus Impaired temperature regulation Fluid and electrolyte abnormalities	Irregular menses Hypoglycemia Mineralocorticoid excess Electrolyte imbalances Dehydration Nephropathy	Diabetes due to obesity
Hematologic	Pancytopenia due to starvation Decreased erythrocyte sedimentation rate	—	—
Pulmonary/mediastinal	—	Aspiration pneumonitis Pneumomediastinum with weight loss or precipitated by vomiting Pneumothorax or rib fractures	—

Data from Walsh JME, Wheat ME, Freund K. Detection, evaluation, and treatment of eating disorders. J Gen Intern Med 2000;15:577–90.

individual and family stature when estimating, particularly for patients with AN. How to calculate IBW is further complicated in the adolescent patient, whereby age-related percentiles need to be taken into consideration in determining what is ideal. A starting point to determine IBW for adults is a BMI of 18 to 19 and for adolescents a BMI in the 50th percentile for age and gender. In premenarchal girls or postmenarchal women experiencing amenorrhea, the goal weight should be adjusted higher to a value where regular menses occurs. Additional goals of treatment are reviewed in **Table 7**.

Table 4 Severity classification of anorexia nervosa	
Mild	BMI $\geq$ 17 kg/m^2
Moderate	BMI 16–16.99 kg/m^2
Severe	BMI 15–15.99 kg/m^2
Extreme	BMI < 15 kg/m^2

Reprinted with permission from the Diagnostic and Statistical Manual of Mental Disorders, Fifth Edition, (Copyright ©2013). American Psychiatric Association. All Rights Reserved.

BULIMIA NERVOSA

BN is characterized by binge eating (eg, eating an amount of food in a short period of time that is much larger than normal) with a feeling of lack of control, followed by compensatory purging behaviors.[10] The full diagnostic criteria are listed in **Table 1**. The lack of emaciation, or being significantly underweight, as well as lack of excessive restrictive behavior separates BN from the binge-eating/purging type of AN; most patients presenting with BN are normal weight or overweight. As with AN patients, BN patients typically have a fear of gaining weight, a strong desire to lose weight, and extreme dissatisfaction with their bodies. BN is associated with young girls, with prevalence highest in young adults. As with AN, it is more common in girls and women than boys and men, with a ratio estimated to be 10:1.[19] The patient interview should include questions about prior trauma, abuse, affective disorders, and bullying.[20]

Menstrual irregularities and amenorrhea can also occur in women with BN. Abnormal laboratory test findings are typically the result of purging behaviors and may include fluid and electrolyte fluctuations. GI issues may be present as the result of laxative abuse. Dental enamel may be damaged from repeatedly induced vomiting.[21] However, as with patients who present with AN, there may be no physical or laboratory test findings supporting the diagnosis. **Table 3** lists medical complications of BN, and **Table 5** lists severity classifications of BN.

Table 5 Severity classification of bulimia nervosa	
Mild	An average of 1–3 episodes of inappropriate compensatory behaviors per week
Moderate	An average of 4–7 episodes of inappropriate compensatory behaviors per week
Severe	An average of 8–13 episodes of inappropriate compensatory behaviors per week
Extreme	An average of 14 or more episodes of inappropriate compensatory behaviors per week

Reprinted with permission from the Diagnostic and Statistical Manual of Mental Disorders, Fifth Edition, (Copyright ©2013). American Psychiatric Association. All Rights Reserved.

BINGE EATING DISORDER

BED is newly categorized in DSM-5. It is characterized by eating much more than normal in a short period of time, accompanied by feelings of lack of control and followed by feelings of disgust or guilt. Patients with BED characteristically eat when not hungry and/or eat until they feel uncomfortably full. These patients typically hide eating behavior and feel shame.

Men are more likely to present with BED than with either AN or BN. Similarly, ethnic groups are as likely as whites to exhibit BED behaviors, in contrast to the other 2 disorders discussed in this article.[22] The condition can begin in adolescence or young adulthood, but also in adulthood. Most patients with the condition have a history of dieting, although the restrictive behavior found in AN is not found in BED. Patients are typically overweight or obese. Risks factors include certain adverse childhood experiences, parental depression, vulnerability to obesity, and repeated exposure to negative comments about shape, weight, and eating (**Tables 6** and **7**).[23]

Table 6 Severity classification of binge eating disorder	
Mild	1–3 binge-eating episodes per week
Moderate	4–7 binge-eating episodes per week
Severe	8–13 binge-eating episodes per week
Extreme	14 or more binge-eating episodes per week

ROLE OF MEDICATIONS

In the absence of any psychiatric comorbidity, there are few pharmacologic options for the treatment of ED. Currently, the only US Food and Drug Administration (FDA) indicated medication for treatment of BN is fluoxetine (daily high dose 60 mg/d), which has shown to decrease the frequency of binge eating and purging[25]; lisdexamfetamine was recently approved by the FDA for treatment of BED.

Off-label uses of novel antipsychotics, medications for attention deficit disorder, antiseizure medications, and other approaches have been tried but are not discussed here.[26] Given the high degree of psychiatric comorbidities in patients with ED, the PCP should be vigilant and screen for affective disorders and other conditions.

LEVELS OF CARE

The American Psychiatric Association has identified 5 levels of care for ED.[24] Level 1, outpatient management, is particularly suited to the PCP. It should be noted that, depending on the physician's practice setting (ie, hospital), comfort level, and available local resources, PCPs can also capably participate in level 2 to 5 care. As described in Practice Guideline for the Treatment of Patients with Eating Disorders, 3rd edition, determinants of levels of care, from outpatient to inpatient hospitalization, are based on 10 criteria: (1) medical status; (2) suicidality; (3) weight as a percentage of IBW; (4) motivation; (5) comorbidities; (6) self-sufficiency in managing appropriate eating behaviors; (7) self-sufficiency in managing excessive exercise; (8) self-sufficiency in controlling purging behavior; (9) environmental stresses or supports; and (10) proximity to treatment facilities. Treatment environments range from (1)

Table 7
Early goals of treatment

	AN	BN	BED
Weight	Restoration to approximately 90% of IBW; increase by 0.5–1.0 pounds a week to (IBW). Adjust target higher if patient postmenarche and still experiencing amenorrhea	Maintenance of weight in range of healthy BMI	Pursue weight loss of obese/overweight patients through reduction in bingeing and maintenance of weight in range of healthy BMI
Medical comorbidities	Reduction in the risk for medical complications as outlined in **Table 3**. Resumption of regular menses in patients with amenorrhea	Reduction in the risk for medical complications as outlined in **Table 3**. Decrease in GI and oropharyngeal symptoms secondary to reduction in purging	Monitor comorbidities related to obesity/overweight
Psychiatric comorbidities	Combination of therapy and medication management	Combination of therapy and medication management	Combination of therapy and medication management
Nutritional rehabilitation and attitude to food	Restore weight, normalize eating patterns, achieve normal perceptions of hunger and satiety[24]	Develop a structured meal plan as a means of reducing the episodes of dietary restriction and the urges to binge and purge[24]	Reduction in reliance for food in managing responses to emotional triggers
Exercise and physical activity	Initial cessation of exercise and nonessential physical activity to conserve calories; when weight restored, can resume physician-guided activity provided net caloric intake supports maintenance of weight	Physician-guided activity to maintain a healthy BMI	Physician-guided activity to maintain a healthy BMI
Purging behaviors	Reduction or cessation in frequency of purging if AN-BP subtype	Reduction or cessation in frequency of purging	—

Adapted from APA Working Group in Eating Disorders. Practice guideline for the treatment of patients with eating disorders, 3rd edition. American Psychiatric Association, 2006.

outpatient; (2) intensive outpatient; (3) full-day outpatient; (4) residential treatment facility; and (5) inpatient hospitalization. Patients who are medically stable, have fair to good motivation to recover, have stable weight of greater than 85% IBW are more likely to be successful in outpatient environments. Obviously, patients who are medically unstable, who express or exhibit suicidal thoughts and behaviors, who suffer from psychiatric comorbidities, and/or who refuse to eat or must be monitored to control bingeing are candidates for hospitalization.

THE EATING DISORDER TREATMENT TEAM

The ideal ED treatment team consists of the triad of physician, therapist, and nutritionist. Each plays a critical role, whose expertise and prominence in the team can shift over time. At steady state, when there are few to no medical complications, the therapist is the lead clinician. Cognitive behavior therapy is the most common, and the most successful, form of counseling, particularly for BN and BED cases.[27] In the setting of medical issues, the physician takes the lead. Given the need for a fluid team, PCPs who care for ED patients should have a therapist and nutritionist with whom they have a good working relationship and who are available for regular consultation. Friends and family can also be integral parts of the treatment team. Patients should be cautioned about pursuing treatment without inclusion of those who can provide a stable and nurturing environment. Given the stigma associated with ED, some prefer the option for "going it alone" because it can provide anonymity and secrecy. Not uncommonly, some patients suspect that the fewer people who know about the treatment plan, the less the treatment plan will need to be followed. Others do not wish to create concern among loved ones. Still others recognize that the structure at home may be a contributing factor to disordered eating. Given the multiple factors involved, the decision to include family in the treatment process is one that requires the physician and patient to be co-decision-makers after a full understanding of the exacerbating and mitigating effect family members can have. Certainly for minors, there is less flexibility in this decision to include or not include family.

THE OFFICE VISIT

Physicians caring for patients with ED need to ensure that their office settings are comfortable for this group, who generally avoid health care providers and who are sensitive to certain imagery and dialogue. Magazines and other reading material in the waiting room should be screened for imagery and subject matter that can prove counterproductive to treatment, including popular press items that stress weight loss, appearance, and so on. Other material, including patient education resources encouraging weight loss, should also be screened for similar mixed messages. Given the heterogeneity of patients seen by the PCP, understandably there are limits to how much can be controlled. Office personnel should be coached to limit comments about appearance that would otherwise seem benign to the non-ED patient (eg, "you look great today"). Scales and mirrors should be removed from the examination room.

To limit the focus on weight alone, individuals with ED, particularly those with weight gain goals, should be discouraged from self-weighing and rely strictly on the weight measured in the provider's office. It may be necessary to remove scales from home and other settings. Weights should be conducted after void, in a gown, on the same scale. Because there is considerable debate about the value of allowing patients to know their weight, the decision needs to be individualized, although most providers prefer blinding patients to weight. Many patients will see any number as too high, so blinding the patient to their weight and indicating progress in less specific terms (eg, "you are on track for weight gain," "your weight is up/down,") may provide relief. The recent widespread adoption of electronic medical records, the increasing focus by payers to record and address BMI for non-ED patients, and improved patient access to his or her own records make the ability to fully blind the patient to weight challenging. If specialists and others are involved, it is likely that they will weigh the patient as part of the general intake process. Patients should be reminded to inform other practitioners that they do not wish to know what they weigh.

WHEN TO REFER

Caring for patients with ED can be a very rewarding process. However, PCPs need to understand that progress can be very slow and sporadic. Unlike weight loss or monitoring improvement based on an abnormal laboratory test value (eg, diabetes with HBa1c), the complexity of ED makes the recovery progress rarely linear. The PCP treating patients with ED should take the following questions into consideration:

- You may be comfortable with patients who are underweight, but are your cross-covering colleagues?
- Do you have a mental health professional and nutritionist with whom you have strong working relationships?
- Can your physical office setting manage the particularities of treating patients with ED?
- Are you comfortable in treating chronic mental health disorders in general?

If the PCP answers no to any of the above questions, then referral may be appropriate. Providers should consider referring to integrated programs. There are many that offer the full spectrum of care from outpatient to inpatient treatment. If a PCP does refer his or her patient, it will be important to continue following the patient's progress regularly. Once patients are discharged from facilities and programs, they will often rely on the PCP to continue the plan. Moreover, the necessity to manage other chronic diseases, including preventive health needs, requires the PCP to remain an integral part of the treatment team during, and especially after, referral to a more comprehensive setting.

REFERENCES

1. Fairburn G, Harrison P. Eating disorder. Lancet 2003;361:407–16.
2. Striegel-Moore H, Dohm FA, Kraemer HC, et al. Eating disorders in white and black women. Am J Psychiatry 2003;160:1326–31.
3. Rosen D. Identification and management of eating disorders in children and adolescents. Pediatrics 2010;126(6):1240–53.
4. American Psychiatric Association. Diagnostic and statistical manual of mental disorders. Washington, DC: American Psychiatric Association; 1952.
5. Lucas AR, Beard CM, O'Fallon WM, et al. 50-year trends in the incidence of anorexia nervosa in Rochester, Minn.: a population-based study. Am J Psychiatry 1991;19(4):681–700.
6. Steinhausen H. The outcome of anorexia nervosa in the 20th century. Am J Psychiatry 2002;159:1284–93.
7. Nicholla DE, Lynn R, Viner RM. Childhood eating disorders: British National Surveillance Study. Br J Psychiatry 2011;198(4):295–301.
8. Schoemaker C. Does early intervention improve the prognosis in anorexia nervosa? A systematic review of the treatment-outcome literature. Int J Eat Disord 1997;21(1):1–15.

9. Tantleff-Dunn S, Barnes RD, Larose JG. It's not just a "woman thing;" the current state of normative discontent. Eat Disord 2011;19(5):392–402.

10. American Psychiatric Association. Diagnostic and statistical manual of mental disorders. 5th edition. Washington, DC: American Psychiatric Association; 2013.

11. Harrington B, Jimmerson M. Initial evaluation, diagnosis, and treatment of anorexia nervosa and bulimia nervosa. Am Fam Physician 2015;91(1):46–52.

12. Solmi F, Hatch SL, Hotopf M, et al. Validation of the SCOFF questionnaire for eating disorders in a multiethnic general population sample. Int J Eat Disord 2015;48(3):312–6.

13. Statistics: Understanding statistics on eating disorders. NEDIC Web site. Available at: http://www.nedic.ca/know-facts/statistics. Accessed July 4, 2015.

14. Crago M, Shisslak CM, Estes LS. Eating disturbances among American minority groups: a review. Int J Eat Disord 1996;19(3):239–48.

15. Katzman D. Medical complications in adolescents with anorexia nervosa: a review of the literature. Int J Eat Disord 2005;37(suppl):s22–59.

16. Walsh JME, Wheat ME, Freund K. Detection, evaluation, and treatment of eating disorders. J Gen Intern Med 2000;15:577–90.

17. Erikesen S. Bone and vitamin D status in patients with anorexia nervosa. Dan Med J 2014;61(11):A4940.

18. Le Grange D, Doyle PM, Swanson SA, et al. Calculation of expected body weight in adolescents with eating disorders. Pediatrics 2012;129(2):e438–46.

19. Hoek HW, van Hoeken D. Review of the prevalence and incidence of eating disorders. Int J Eat Disord 2003;34:4.

20. Kaltiala-Heino R, Rimpela M, Rantanen P, et al. Bullying at school—an indicator of adolescents at risk for mental disorders. J Adolesc 2000;23(6):661–74.

21. Mitchell JE, Crow S. Medical complications of anorexia nervosa and bulimia nervosa. Curr Opin Psychiatry 2006;19(4):438–43.

22. Striegel-Moore R. Epidemiology of binge eating disorder. Int J Eat Disord 2003; 34(Suppl):S19–29.

23. Fairburn C, Doll HA, Welch SL, et al. Risk factors for binge eating disorder: a community-based, case-control study. Arch Gen Psychiatry 1998;55(5):425–32.

24. American Psychiatric Association. Practice guideline for the treatment of patients with eating disorders. 3rd edition. Washington, DC: American Psychiatric Association; 2006.

25. Freeman C. Drug treatment for bulimia nervosa. Neuropsychobiology 1998;37: 72–9.

26. Hay PH, Claudino AM. Clinical psychopharmacology of eating disorders: a research update. Int J Neuropsychopharmacol 2012;15(2):209–22.

27. National Collaborating Centre for Mental Health (UK). Eating Disorders: Core Interventions in the Treatment and Management of Anorexia Nervosa, Bulimia Nervosa and Related Eating Disorders. Leicester (UK): British Psychological Society; 2004.

Childhood Sexual Abuse

Identification, Screening, and Treatment Recommendations in Primary Care Settings

Rochelle F. Hanson, PhD[a],*, Cristin S. Adams, DO[b]

KEYWORDS

- Childhood sexual abuse • Sexual abuse screening • Childhood PTSD
- Trauma-focused cognitive behavioral therapy (TF-CBT) • Sexual victimization

KEY POINTS

- Childhood sexual abuse (CSA) poses a significant risk to children, both in terms of acute reactions as well as the increased likelihood of long-term physical and mental health problems.
- Available data consistently indicate that girls and adolescents are at a higher risk for sexual victimization; because of barriers related to screening and disclosure, current epidemiologic evidence is likely an underestimation of the actual incidence and prevalence of CSA.
- Use of validated screening tools and targeted clinical examination in the primary care setting can help identify children who may benefit from further evaluation to determine treatment needs.
- Given the paucity of data in the pediatric population, the use of medications to treat trauma-related symptoms, such as posttraumatic stress disorder, is reserved for refractory cases and patients with comorbid diagnoses for which pharmacologic management is widely accepted.
- Because of their role in children's health care, primary care providers should provide guidance for victims and their families and be knowledgeable about their mandated responsibilities for reporting suspected abuse.

The authors have no financial or commercial conflicts of interest to disclose.
[a] Department of Psychiatry and Behavioral Sciences, National Crime Victims Research and Treatment Center, Medical University of South Carolina, 67 President Street, MSC861, Charleston, SC 29425, USA; [b] PGY-3 Trident/MUSC Family Medicine Residency, Department of Family Medicine, Medical University of South Carolina, 135 Rutledge Avenue, Charleston, SC 29425, USA
* Corresponding author.
E-mail address: hansonrf@musc.edu

INTRODUCTION
Definition of Childhood Sexual Abuse

The National Child Traumatic Stress Network (www.nctsn.org) defines childhood sexual abuse (CSA) as "any interaction between a child and an adult (or another child) in which the child is used for sexual stimulation of the perpetrator or an observer."[1] Sexual abuse can involve touching as well as nontouching behaviors, including voyeurism, exhibitionism, or exposing the child to pornography. It is important to recognize that not all children experience physical force; but instead, offenders may use a variety of coercive, manipulative, and deceptive tactics to engage children in sexual activity and reduce the likelihood of disclosure.

Prevalence and Incidence of Childhood Sexual Abuse

CSA poses a significant risk to children, both in terms of acute reactions as well as the increased likelihood of long-term physical and mental health problems.[2–4] As a consequence, CSA and other forms of maltreatment present a substantial and costly public health concern.[5] In a recent review of epidemiologic studies of trauma in childhood, Saunders and Adams[6] provided information on prevalence and incidence of trauma, challenges to understanding the existing epidemiologic data, and recommendations for clinicians regarding best practice for screening of trauma and its impact. Interested readers are referred to the publication for further details.

Based on recent national data, between 8% and 12% of youths have experienced at least one sexual assault in their lifetime.[6] This percentage is in comparison with approximately

- 9% to 19% who have experienced physical abuse by a caregiver or physical assault
- 38% to 70% who have witnessed serious community violence
- 10% who have witnessed serious violence between caregivers
- 20% who have lost a family member or friend to homicide

Data from the National Survey of Children's Exposure to Violence[7] (NatSCEV), which included a nationally representative sample of 4000 children aged 0 to 17 years, indicated that 2.0% of girls experienced sexual assault or sexual abuse within the study year (2013–2014), whereas 4.6% of girls aged 14 to 17 years experienced sexual victimization within the 1-year period.[8,9] Youths rarely report exposure to a single event; rather, exposure to multiple types of trauma, referred to as *poly-victimization*, is very common, with prevalence rates ranging from 20% to 48%.[10] Available data consistently indicate that certain factors, such as sex and age, confer added risk for sexual victimization. For example, data from the NatSCEV indicated that girls were 1.5 times more likely than boys to report at least 1 episode of sexual victimization within the past year. Adolescents are at higher risk as compared with younger children.[8] For example, in the National Survey of Adolescents[11,12] (NSA) and NSA-Replication[13,14] (NSA-R), 8% of adolescents reported at least one sexual victimization in their lifetime, with significantly higher rates for girls versus boys (13% vs 3%, respectively). Taken together, available data indicate that girls have a 3 to 4 times greater risk for sexual victimization than boys.

Another important issue, particularly for female adolescents, is drug- or alcohol-facilitated sexual assault. McCauley and colleagues[15] analyzed data from the NSA-R and found that 2% of interviewed girls reported that they had been sexually assaulted while incapacitated because of drugs or alcohol.

An important caveat to any of the available epidemiologic data is that any estimate of sexual abuse or sexual assault is likely to be an underestimate because of several factors[7] (**Box 1**):

- Fear, shame, or embarrassment to report on the part of the victim
- Reliance on reported rates (such as those reported to law enforcement or child protective services), because few sexual assaults are actually officially reported to authorities
- Considerable variability in methodology across studies, such as differences in the definitions of sexual victimization and the types of screening questions used to obtain these data

SCREENING FOR CHILDHOOD SEXUAL ABUSE HISTORY AND RELATED SYMPTOMS
To Screen or Not to Screen?

The US Preventive Services Task Force has determined that "current evidence is insufficient"[16] to recommend specific preventive interventions in the primary care setting (http://www.uspreventiveservicestaskforce.org/). This determination results in a lack of consensus regarding the use of universal screening for children. There are, however, compelling reasons to encourage some type of brief screening as part of routine care. First, research studies indicate that more parents (94%–96%) seek services for their children through primary care settings, compared with only 4% to 33% of parents directly seeking mental health services.[17] Second, for many children, the primary care provider may be their only contact with a professional who has the knowledge, expertise, and resources to provide needed assistance. Thus, primary care settings can offer a unique opportunity to bridge mental and physical health services; use of a brief instrument to screen for history of abuse and abuse-related symptoms increases the likelihood that children are identified and can be referred for further evaluation and treatment when warranted.[18–21]

Whether or not universal screening is used, it is important for primary care providers to be aware of potential signs or symptoms of sexual abuse.[22] These signs and symptoms may include visible signs of distress at the time of the office visit, such as anxiety about separation from a caregiver, refusal to get undressed, or unwillingness to be examined by the provider. Caregivers may report concerns about the child's behavior, such as nightmares, difficulty sleeping alone, a sudden or increased fear of the dark, bed-wetting for a child who was previously toilet trained, sadness, withdrawal, irritability, and anger outbursts. Children and/or caregivers may also report physical symptoms, such as headaches, stomachaches, and fatigue. Additionally, children may display sexual knowledge, sexual language, or engage in sexual behaviors that are inappropriate for their age. If any of these behaviors are present, further assessment is warranted.

Screening for Childhood Sexual Abuse History

Noted barriers to the use of formal instruments to screen for CSA or other traumatic events in primary care settings include limited time and resources. In response to

---

Box 1
Reasons for underestimating rates of sexual assault

- Fear, shame, embarrassment to report
- Reliance on reported rates because few sexual assaults are actually reported to authorities
- Variability in methodology (eg, differences in definitions; differences in types of screening)

these legitimate concerns, self-report measures, such as the Trauma Screen developed by the Harborview Center for Sexual Assault or the Trauma Events Screening Inventory for Children,[23,24] can be completed by the child and/or caregiver in the waiting room and then reviewed during the face-to-face appointment time. This procedure is predicated on (1) having a private area where these measures can be completed and (2) the practitioner taking the time to review the information with patients. However, because CSA is often accompanied by secrecy as well as negative attributions, such as shame, self-blame, guilt, and embarrassment, self-report measures may not result in disclosure. If other risk factors (eg, caregiver refusal to leave the child or child's fear of being undressed in front of the practitioner) or overt signs of abuse are present, direct (and, if possible, private) questioning of the child should be considered. Referral to a professional with expertise in conducting forensic evaluations (ie, to make an informed, objective determination about the likelihood of abuse) may be advisable.

As discussed by Saunders and Adams,[7] the best, and most valid, methods to screen for a history of sexual victimization include

- Use of clarifying introductions to help orient the respondent
- Avoidance of single-item gate questions (eg, Have you ever been sexually abused?)
- Use of several screening questions to provide multiple opportunities for the respondent
- Use of behaviorally specific screening questions
- Avoidance of vague summary terms, such as *abuse* or *trauma*

However, this type of comprehensive screening may be impractical in a busy primary care setting. Thus, use of a single gate question, such as the one recommended by Cohen and colleagues[19] (*"Since the last time I saw you, has anything really scary or upsetting happened to you or your family?"*[19]), provides some indication of which children may need further screening or assessment.

Screening for Abuse-Related Symptoms

As noted earlier, comprehensive assessment presents feasibility challenges for most primary care settings. However, use of brief tools, designed to assess for symptoms most common among abused children, including posttraumatic stress disorder (PTSD), depression, anxiety, or sexualized behaviors,[22] present a viable option, particularly for those children evidencing potential signs of abuse and/or situations whereby caregivers express specific concerns. **Table 1** provides an overview of some brief instruments to assess for trauma-related symptoms and other behavioral or emotional problems that can result from CSA. For a detailed review, please refer to Wherry and colleagues.[21]

The University of California, Los Angeles Posttraumatic Stress Disorder Reaction Index[25,26] and the Child Posttraumatic Symptom Scale[27] are both reliable and valid measures of PTSD symptoms for children and adolescents. The Moods and Feelings Questionnaire[28] offers a brief screen for depression, whereas Screen for Childhood Anxiety Related Emotional Disorders (SCARED)[29] measures anxiety symptoms and provides a brief screen for posttraumatic stress symptoms. Although not trauma specific, the Pediatric Symptom Checklist-17[30] is a brief caregiver-completed measure of internalizing (depression, sadness), externalizing (behavioral), and attentional problems. The Children's Sexual Behavior Inventory (CSBI)[31,32] is a 38-item caregiver-completed measure to assess sexual behaviors in children aged 2 to 12 years. The CSBI yields a total score as well as 2 additional subscales. Research has

Table 1
Screening instruments

	Instrument	Author	Brief Description	Clinical Cutoff
Trauma history screen	Harborview Trauma Screen	Harborview Center for Sexual Assault and Traumatic Stress	14 Items to assess exposure to variety of potentially traumatic events as well as life threat, fear someone else would die or be seriously harmed; feelings of helplessness, shame, or disgust	No cutoff; measure of exposure to trauma
	Trauma Events Screening Inventory for Children (TESI) (4 y and older)	Ribbe,[23] 1996; Ippen et al,[24] 2002	14-Item clinician-administered interview to assess variety of potentially traumatic events; includes items to assess DSM-IV PTSD criterion A (NOTE: Child self-report and caregiver report forms are also available.)	No cutoff; measure of exposure to trauma
Posttraumatic stress symptoms	UCLA Posttraumatic Stress Disorder Reaction Index (7–17 y)	Pynoos et al,[25] 1998; Steinberg et al,[26] 2004	17 Items to measure DSM-IV symptoms of posttraumatic stress and 2 items to measure associated symptoms of guilt and fear of event's recurrence	—
	Child Posttraumatic Symptom Scale (CPSS) (8–18 y)	Foa et al,[27] 2001	17 Items to measure DSM-IV posttraumatic stress symptoms and 7 items to measure functional impairment	Total score of ≥12
Other behavioral/ emotional problems	Moods and Feelings Questionnaire (MFQ) (7–18 y)	Angold et al,[28] 1987	13-Item measure of depressive symptoms	Total score of ≥11
	Pediatric Symptom Checklist-17 (PSC-17) (caregiver completed)	Gardner et al,[30] 1999	17-Item caregiver-completed measure of overall problems, internalizing (sadness, anxiety), externalizing (behavior problems), and attentional problems	Total score of ≥15
	Screen for Childhood Anxiety Related Emotional Disorders (SCARED) Brief Assessment of Anxiety and PTSD Symptoms (7–17)	Muris et al,[64] 2000	5 Items measure anxiety; 4 items measure PTSD (mainly intrusion symptoms)	Anxiety: ≥3 PTSD: ≥6
	Child Sexual Behavior Inventory (CSBI) (caregiver completed for children aged 2–12 y)	Friedrich,[31] 1998; Friedrich et al,[32] 2001	38 Items to assess children who have been or may have been sexually abused Yields total score and 2 subscale scores: developmentally related sexual behaviors and sexual abuse–specific items	Normative scores by age and sex

Abbreviations: DSM-IV, Diagnostic and Statistical Manual for Mental Disorders (Fourth Edition); PTSD, posttraumatic stress disorder; UCLA, University of California, Los Angeles.
Data from Refs.[23–28,30–32,64]

demonstrated that sexually abused children are reported to exhibit greater frequencies of sexual behaviors than normative or psychiatric outpatient samples. However, sexual behavior problems are not a definitive sign of CSA. Alternative explanations include the child's accidental exposure to sexually explicit materials, family nudity, or unintentional exposure to parents' sexual activity.[32]

For any of these measures, scores in the clinical range would warrant further inquiry and potential referral for a more extensive evaluation. As an additional caveat, caregiver and child reports may yield discrepant results. In cases whereby the child, but not the caregiver, report abuse, it is important that the child's disclosure not be discounted and instead leads to further inquiry and possible referral for a more comprehensive evaluation.

Some additional caveats related to screening are important to note:

- In the case of CSA in particular, children may not acknowledge the abuse occurred or may be too ashamed to report.
- Young children may not understand or have the verbal or cognitive capacity to recognize that their experience was abusive, making it particularly important to collect information from other sources, such as a caregiver, when possible. If there are concerns about the caregiver, it may be necessary to seek additional, collateral reporters, such as school or day care personnel.
- Certain symptoms, behavioral problems, and disorders may preexist or be exacerbated by abuse.[21] However, there is no empirical basis to conclude that child abuse in and of itself causes severe psychiatric problems.
- As noted in the American Academy of Child and Adolescent Psychiatry's (AACAP, 2010) "Practice Parameter for the Assessment and Treatment of Children and Adolescents with Posttraumatic Stress Disorder,"[33] practitioners need to consider differential diagnoses when assessing for abuse-related symptoms. Symptoms of PTSD can mirror those of other psychiatric disorders. For example, visual hallucinations may actually be re-experiencing of events through flashbacks rather than psychosis. Emotion dysregulation may stem from abuse-related fear and anxiety rather than bipolar disorder. Panic symptoms may be triggered by an abuse-related cue or reminder rather than reflecting panic disorder. Concentration problems or hyperactivity may be symptomatic of PTSD hyperarousal symptoms rather than attention-deficit/hyperactivity disorder (**Table 2**).

Lastly, providers should not assume that all sexually abused children have symptoms related to their abuse experience. Although some may develop symptoms later on, not all will develop long-term significant problems related to their abuse. In fact, one early study indicated that approximately 25% of individuals with a CSA history did not meet the criteria for any adjustment problems.[34] Thus, assuming that all

Table 2	
Posttraumatic stress disorder can mirror symptoms of other psychiatric disorders	
Symptoms of Other Disorders	**PTSD**
Visual hallucinations (psychosis)	Re-experiencing symptoms (eg, flashbacks)
Emotion dysregulation (bipolar disorder)	Abuse-related fear and anxiety
Panic symptoms (panic disorder)	Abuse-related trigger
Concentration problems/hyperactivity (attention-deficit/hyperactivity disorder)	Hyperarousal

children who experience abuse are traumatized can result in misdiagnosis and inappropriate referrals for treatment.[21]

TREATMENT OPTIONS
Pharmacologic Strategies

Although no specific protocols exist regarding pharmacologic interventions for CSA victims, there have been recommendations made for children experiencing related PTSD (**Table 3**). The "Practice Parameter for the Assessment and Treatment of Children and Adolescents with Posttraumatic Stress Disorder"[33] includes 2 recommendations regarding pharmacologic treatment based on expert opinion:

- Selective serotonin reuptake inhibitors (SSRIs) can be considered for the treatment of children and adolescents with PTSD.
- Medications other than SSRIs may be considered for youths with PTSD.

These parameters specify that pharmacotherapy may be considered only when an adequate trial of evidence-based psychotherapy alone is ineffective. Medications should serve as an element of a comprehensive treatment plan, as an adjunct to psychotherapy; comorbid psychiatric diagnoses should be treated simultaneously. However, careful review of medication adverse effects and consideration of risks versus benefits of different treatment regimens are particularly important given the limited body of evidence and lack of long-term data in this field. Next (and listed in **Table 3**) is a brief overview of the primary pharmacologic agents for children with trauma-related symptoms, as recommended in the AACAP's practice parameters.[33]

Selective serotonin reuptake inhibitors

SSRIs are the most widely prescribed class of medications in childhood PTSD because of their favorable side-effect profile and target of multiple symptoms. The limited research that exists is promising regarding their efficacy. In a pilot randomized controlled trial (RCT) comparing Trauma-Focused Cognitive Behavioral Therapy (TF-CBT; an evidence-based mental health treatment approach; see next section) plus sertraline with TF-CBT plus placebo, children with sexual abuse–related PTSD symptoms showed improved clinical outcomes in both groups but greater improvement in Child Global Assessment Scale ratings in the TF-CBT plus sertraline group.[35]

Citalopram has been shown to improve symptoms in adolescents with severe PTSD[36] and results in similar improvement for adults with PTSD.[37] However, another RCT showed no difference in PTSD symptom improvement in children treated with sertraline and placebo.[38] Therefore, TF-CBT alone remains the preferred initial treatment.

Table 3
Pharmacologic agents

Medication Class	Target Symptoms
Selective serotonin reuptake inhibitors	First line for all symptom clusters
Central adrenergic blockers	Hyperarousal
Beta-adrenergic blockers	Hyperarousal
Tricyclic antidepressants	Depression or anxiety
Antiepileptics	Mood dysregulation
Atypical antipsychotics	Mood dysregulation or psychosis with comorbid psychiatric diagnoses

Central alpha-adrenergic agonists

Alpha-adrenergic agonists have shown some benefit, particularly in targeting hyper-arousal symptoms associated with PTSD. Nighttime use of guanfacine showed improvement in all symptom severity measures of children with PTSD particularly impacting anxiety, traumatic stress, and functional impairment.[39] Preschool-aged children with PTSD treated with clonidine showed reductions in aggression, insomnia, and hyperarousal.[40]

Beta-adrenergic blockers

With increased adrenergic tone implicated in some symptom clusters of PTSD, adren-ergic blocking agents have theoretic appeal and may be effective. In a pilot study of children with PTSD due to physical and/or sexual abuse treated with propranolol, Famularo and colleagues[41] found symptoms improved during the treatment period but regressed after medication withdrawal.

Tricyclic antidepressants

Tricyclic antidepressants may be considered as a treatment option when depressive or anxious symptoms predominate in childhood PTSD, but potential cardiac side ef-fects require caution and limit use. In a prospective study of children hospitalized for thermal injury with associated acute stress disorder (ASD), those treated with imip-ramine had fewer ASD symptoms and were less likely to develop PTSD.[42]

Antiepileptics

Antiepileptics are often used for mood stabilization and have a potential role when symptoms of mood dysregulation prevail or appropriate coexisting conditions are pre-sent. A prospective study of child CSA victims treated with carbamazepine showed improvement in PTSD symptoms, with more than half having comorbid psychiatric di-agnoses for which they were receiving additional psychotropic medications.[43]

Atypical antipsychotics

Given their side-effect profile and related concern with long-term use, these agents should only be considered for extreme presentations or when other psychiatric comorbidities exist. An open trial of boys with severe PTSD and multiple other psychi-atric diagnoses showed improvement in most subjects treated with risperidone.[44]

Nonpharmacologic Strategies

Trauma-focused mental health treatments

As discussed, not all children who experience abuse will develop problems either acutely or long-term. However, given the increased risk, it is imperative that children have access to trauma-focused, evidence-based treatments (EBTs) (Note: For purposes of this article, EBTs or empirically supported treatments are those that have been rigorously evaluated and found to be efficacious in RCTs.) To date, the most widely disseminated and effective intervention for children exposed to trauma is TF-CBT.[45–49] As Black and colleagues[49] concluded in their review: "TF-CBT is the most studied, the most endorsed, of all of the treatments for trauma-related symp-toms among children and adolescents. It is well established and research has effec-tively demonstrated that it reduces symptoms of trauma."[49(pp200)] Cary and McMillen[46] note that TF-CBT received the highest classification rating for levels of ev-idence and effectiveness from the following sources: (1) California Evidence-Based Clearinghouse for Child Welfare (www.cebc4cw.org), (2) Kaufman Best Practices Proj-ect (www.chadwickcenter.org/Kauffman/kauffman.htm), and (3) Substance Abuse

Mental Health Services Administration National Registry of Evidence-Based Practices and Programs.

TF-CBT is a structured, time-limited (ie, 12–20 therapy sessions) intervention that includes specific components to provide education about trauma and its impact, enhance relaxation and coping skills to manage abuse-related symptoms, and enable children to discuss their abuse in a detailed fashion in order to process inaccurate or unhelpful thinking patterns related to the abuse. Joint parent-child sessions may facilitate sharing and open communication about the traumatic events and improve parenting skills to manage problematic child behaviors that may have preexisted but are now exacerbated by the abuse. For further information about TF-CBT, readers are referred to Hanson and Jobe-Shields[50] and Pollio and colleagues.[51]

LONG-TERM PHYSICAL AND MENTAL HEALTH EFFECTS OF CHILDHOOD SEXUAL ABUSE

The potential long-term impact of CSA is highly variable, and it is generally accepted that no single presentation or syndrome exists. Not all children who experience CSA will develop long-term sequelae, and certain protective factors exist (eg, positive coping strategies, stable living situation, social support, caregiver support).[34,52] A landmark study[22] found that the extent of symptoms experienced by CSA victims was affected by factors, including penetration, duration and frequency of the abuse, use of force, the relationship of the perpetrator to the child, and maternal support. Two-thirds of victims in this study demonstrated recovery during the first 12 to 18 months. Poly-victimization (ie, exposure to multiple traumatic events) is a recognized phenomenon[10]; but when controlling for nonsexual-abuse trauma, CSA still seems to significantly impact youth[10] and adult symptoms.[53]

Regarding long-term effects of CSA,[54] aside from chronic PTSD, the most frequently related diagnoses/symptoms seem to be impaired sense of self, impaired interpersonal functioning, cognitive distortions (eg, helpless/hopelessness, impaired trust, self-blame, low self-esteem), emotional distress (depression, anxiety, anger), and avoidance (dissociation, substance abuse, suicidal ideation and attempts) (**Table 4**).

Although psychological findings may predominate, there have been links to adverse physical outcomes associated with CSA. The Adverse Child Experiences (ACEs) Study,[55] an ongoing prospective study involving more than 17,000 participants, is examining the relationship between ACEs (eg, abuse, neglect, and household dysfunction), physical health, and cause of death. An association exists between ACEs and health-related quality of life, and an increased number of ACEs correlates with poor health outcomes (eg, alcoholism, chronic obstructive pulmonary disease, depression, fetal death, ischemic heart disease, liver disease, and sexually

Table 4	
Long-term effects of childhood sexual abuse	
Effect	**Examples**
Impaired sense of self	Poor self-esteem
Impaired interpersonal functioning	Poor social skills
Cognitive distortions	Helplessness, hopelessness, impaired trust, self-blame, guilt
Emotional distress	Depression, anxiety, anger
Avoidance	Dissociation, substance abuse, suicide

transmitted diseases). ACEs are associated with behaviors that may adversely affect health, including illicit drug use, smoking, multiple sexual partners, intimate partner violence, and unintended pregnancy.

The concept of sexual revictimization in adulthood is a well-described consequence of CSA, with potentiating factors, including engagement in high-risk behaviors, such as substance use and risky sexual behaviors. Primary care clinicians must be aware of this issue to guide continued surveillance throughout the lifespan.[56]

ANTICIPATORY GUIDANCE

Targeted anticipatory guidance regarding CSA should be part of the well-child or adolescent examination. The AAP recommends that young children be educated about their private parts and what constitutes appropriate versus inappropriate touching.[57] Discussion about normal sexual behavior should begin in preschool,[58] and discussion of ok and not ok touch may be helpful to incorporate into preventative visits at this time.[59] Parents should be encouraged to help their children, from an early age, refer to their genitals with anatomically correct terms to make identification of inappropriate actions more likely. Well visits for teens should assess for sexual activity and any concern for abuse or coercion. History should include the ages of sexual partners, in case age-gaps necessitate reporting.[57] Caregivers should be aware that most sexual abuse occurs by someone known to the child; thus, caution should always be used when leaving a child alone with another individual. Because perpetrators often hold positions of influence (ie, teachers, relatives, coaches), victims may blame themselves or may develop a distorted view of authority. Children should be taught to understand the difference between being respectful to adults and giving indiscriminate consent to any behaviors that make them feel uncomfortable. Caregivers should grant permission for children to leave situations that make them uncomfortable and to seek out a trusted adult. An example for how to share this information with children is, "If someone does something to you or makes you do something that doesn't seem right, it is OK to say 'No' and tell me, no matter who that person is."[60]

If abuse is disclosed, the response received by the child can have a lasting impact. Thus, projecting a calm, protective demeanor without extensive repetitive questioning and with reassurance to the victim that it is not his or her fault is of utmost importance.[61,62] CSA is a sensitive and subsequently challenging subject to approach; but by being open and nonjudgmental, primary care providers can provide guidance to families that may prevent abuse, identify victims, and improve outcomes.

MANDATED REPORTING

Physicians are mandated reporters of suspected child abuse or neglect in all states and the District of Columbia. State statutes include protection for reporters to maintain confidentiality, but thorough documentation facilitates protection of the victim and the provider. It is important to note that suspicion of abuse, not proof, is required for reporting. Further details, including what entities to inform, elements to include in reports, and penalties on failure to report, vary by state. Readers are encouraged to familiarize themselves with their state-specific guidelines summarized in the following document: https//www.childwelfare.gov/pubPDFs/manda.pdf.

SUMMARY AND DISCUSSION

Primary care physicians have a potential role in the care of CSA victims at any point in their trajectory; thus, it is important to have an understanding of the epidemiology, diagnosis, treatment, and potential sequelae of CSA. CSA is underreported and, thus, underestimated in the general population. Artful conductance of clinical history and examination by the primary care physician in screening for sexual abuse and other trauma are crucial, and one must recognize the separate role of the forensic examination that should be undertaken only with specialized training. Anticipatory guidance may help educate patients and families on prevention and coping with CSA. The use of validated screening methods may be limited by time in the primary care setting; but brief screens are available to facilitate disclosure, identification, and appropriate referrals when warranted. The highly variable presentation of CSA victims is important to consider when evaluating and treating patients in the primary care setting. From a medicolegal standpoint, it is prudent to be aware of state-specific reporting mandates.

Both PTSD and ASD are recognized as Axis I diagnoses associated with CSA. Both have been updated for inclusion in the *Diagnostic and Statistical Manual of Mental Disorders* (Fifth Edition).[63] In the absence of contraindications, TF-CBT is the first-line treatment of victims of CSA. Medications may be considered in refractory cases or with comorbid psychiatric diagnoses, with SSRIs being first line. Although not universally experienced, the potential psychological and physical impact of CSA, in addition to the increased risk for revictimization, requires attention from providers in all spheres of primary care.

REFERENCES

1. National Child Traumatic Stress Network Child Sexual Abuse Committee (2009). Caring for Kids: What parents need to know about sexual abuse. Los Angeles, CA & Durham, NC: National Center for Child Traumatic Stress.

2. Hanson RF, Borntrager CF, Self-Brown S, et al. Relations among gender, violence exposure, and mental health: the National Survey of Adolescents. Am J Orthopsychiatry 2008;78:313–21.

3. McLaughlin KA, Koenen KC, Hill ED, et al. Trauma exposure and posttraumatic stress disorder in a national sample of adolescents. J Am Acad Child Adolesc Psychiatry 2013;52(8):815–30.

4. Walsh K, Danielson CK, McCauley JL, et al. National prevalence of posttraumatic stress disorder among sexually revictimized adolescent, college, and adult household-residing women. Arch Gen Psychiatry 2012;69(90):935–42.

5. Fang X, Brown DS, Florence CS, et al. The economic burden of child maltreatment in the United States and implications for prevention. Child Abuse Negl 2012;36(2):156–65.

6. Saunders BE, Adams ZA. Epidemiology of traumatic experiences in childhood. Child Adolesc Psychiatr Clin N Am 2013;23:167–84.

7. Saunders BE, Kilpatrick DG, Hanson RF, et al. Prevalence, case characteristics, and long-term psychological correlates of child rape among women: a national survey. Child Maltreat 1999;4:187–200.

8. Finkelhor D, Turner H, Ormrod R, et al. Violence, abuse, and crime exposure in a national sample of children and youth. Pediatrics 2009;124:1411–23.

9. Finkelhor D, Turner H, Shattuck T, et al. Prevalence of childhood exposure to violence, crime, and abuse: results from the National Survey of Children's Exposure to Violence. JAMA Pediatr 2015;169(8):746–54.

10. Finkelhor D, Ormrod R, Turner H. Polyvictimization and trauma in a national cohort. Dev Psychopathol 2007;19:149–66.

11. Kilpatrick DG, Saunders BE, Smith DW. Youth victimization: prevalence and implications. Washington, DC: National Institute of Justice; 2003 (Research in brief) (NCJ 194972).
12. Kilpatrick DG, Saunders BE. Prevalence and consequences of child victimization: results from the National Survey of Adolescents, final report. Washington, DC: U.S. Department of Justice; 1997.
13. Wolitzky-Taylor KB, Ruggiero KJ, McCart MR. Has adolescent suicidality decreased in the United States? Data from two national samples of adolescents interviewed in 1995 and 2005. J Clin Child Adolesc Psychol 2010;39:64–76.
14. McCart MR, Zajac K, Danielson CK. Interpersonal victimization, posttraumatic stress disorder, and change in adolescent substance use prevalence over a ten-year period. J Clin Child Adolesc Psychol 2011;40:136–43.
15. McCauley JL, Conoscenti L, Ruggiero KJ. Prevalence and correlates of drug/alcohol-facilitated and incapacitated sexual assault in a national representative sample of adolescent girls. J Clin Child Adolesc Psychol 2009;38:295–300.
16. U.S. Preventive Services Task Force. Final Recommendation Statement: Child Maltreatment: Primary Care Interventions; 2013. Available at: http://www.uspreventiveservicestaskforce.org/Page/Document/RecommendationStatementFinal/child-maltreatment-primary-care-interventions. Accessed February 26, 2016.
17. Guevara J, Lozano P, Wickizer T, et al. Utilization and cost of health care services for children with attention deficit/hyperactivity disorder. Pediatrics 2001;108(1):71–8.
18. Felitti VJ, Anda RF, Nordenberg D, et al. Relationship of childhood abuse and household dysfunction to many of the leading causes of death in adults: the Adverse Childhood Experiences (ACE) study. Am J Prev Med 1998;14:245–58.
19. Cohen JA, Kelleher KJ, Mannarino AP. The role of pediatric providers. Arch Pediatr Adolesc Med 2008;16:447–52.
20. Briggs EC, Fairbank JA, Greeson JKP, et al. Links between child and adolescent trauma exposure and service use histories in a national clinic-referred sample. Psychol Trauma 2012;5(2):101–9.
21. Wherry JM, Briggs-King E, Hanson RF. Psychosocial assessment in child maltreatment. In: Reece RM, Hanson RF, Sargent J, editors. Treatment of child abuse: common ground for mental health, medical, and legal practitioners. 2nd edition. Baltimore (MD): The Johns Hopkins University Press; 2014. p. 12–30.
22. Kendall-Tackett K, Williams LM, Finkelhor D. Impact of sexual abuse on children: a review and synthesis of recent empirical studies. Psychol Bull 1993;113:1164–80.
23. Ribbe D. Psychometric review of traumatic event screening instrument for children (TESI-C). In: Stamm BH, editor. Measurement of stress, trauma, and adaptation. Lutherville (MD): Sidran Press; 1996. p. 386–7.
24. Ippen CG, Ford J, Racusin R, et al. Traumatic events screening inventory - parent report revised. VA's National Center for PTSD. 2002.
25. Pynoos R, Rodriguez N, Steinberg A, et al. UCLA PTSD index trauma screen for DSM-IV. Los Angeles (CA): UCLA Trauma Psychiatry Service; 1998.
26. Steinberg AM, Brymer MJ, Decker KB, et al. The University of California at Los Angeles post-traumatic stress disorder reaction index. Curr Psychiatry Rep 2004;6:96–100.
27. Foa EB, Johnson KM, Feeny NC, et al. The Child PTSD Symptom Scale: a preliminary examination of its psychometric properties. J Clin Child Psychol 2001;30:376–84.

28. Angold A, Costello EJ, Messer SC, et al. The development of a short question-naire for use in epidemiological studies of depression in children and adoles-cents. International Journal of Methods in Psychiatric Research 1995;5:237–49.

29. Birmaher B, Khetarpal S, Brent D, et al. The screen for child anxiety related emotional disorders (SCARED): scale construction and psychometric character-istics. J Am Acad Child Adolesc Psychiatry 1997;36(4):545–53.

30. Gardner W, Murphy M, Childs G. The PSC-17: a brief pediatric symptom checklist with psychosocial problem subscales. A report from PROS and ASPN. Ambul Child Health 1999;5:225.

31. Friedrich WN. The child sexual behavior inventory professional manual. Odessa (FL): Psychological Assessment Resources; 1998.

32. Friedrich WN, Fisher JL, Dittner CA, et al. Child sexual behavior inventory: norma-tive, psychiatric, and sexual abuse comparisons. Child Maltreat 2001;6(1):37–49.

33. Cohen JA, Bukstein O, Benson SR, et al. Practice parameter for the assessment and treatment of children and adolescents with posttraumatic stress disorder. J Am Acad Child Adolesc Psychiatry 2010;49:414–30.

34. Lynskey MT, Fergusson DM. Factors protecting against the development of adjustment difficulties in young adults exposed to childhood sexual abuse. Child Abuse Negl 1997;21:1177–90.

35. Cohen JA, Mannarino AP, Perel JM, et al. A pilot randomized controlled trial of combined trauma-focused CBT and sertraline for childhood PTSD symptoms. J Am Acad Child Adolesc Psychiatry 2007;46:811–9.

36. Seedat S, Lockhat R, Kaminer D, et al. An open trial of citalopram in adolescents with post-traumatic stress disorder. Int Clin Psychopharmacol 2001;16:21.

37. Seedat S, Stein DJ, Ziervogel C, et al. Comparison of response to a selective se-rotonin reuptake inhibitor in children, adolescents, and adults with posttraumatic stress disorder. J Child Adolesc Psychopharmacol 2002;12:37–46.

38. Robb AS, Cueva JE, Sporn J, et al. Sertraline treatment of children and adoles-cents with posttraumatic stress disorder: A double-blind, placebo-controlled trial. J Child Adolesc Psychopharmacol 2010;20(6):463–71.

39. Connor DF, Grasso DJ, Slivinsky MD, et al. An open-label study of guanfacine extended release for traumatic stress related symptoms in children and adoles-cents. J Child Adolesc Psychopharmacol 2013;23:244–51.

40. Harmon RJ, Riggs PD. Clonidine for posttraumatic stress disorder in preschool children. J Am Acad Child Adolesc Psychiatry 1996;35:1247–9.

41. Famularo R, Kinscherff R, Fenton T. Propranolol treatment for childhood posttrau-matic stress disorder, acute type. A pilot study. Am J Dis Child 1988;142:1244–7.

42. Robert R, Blakeney PE, Villarreal C, et al. Imipramine treatment in pediatric burn patients with symptoms of acute stress disorder: a pilot study. J Am Acad Child Adolesc Psychiatry 1999;38:873–82.

43. Looff D, Grimley P, Kuller F, et al. Carbamazepine for PTSD. J Am Acad Child Adolesc Psychiatry 1995;34:703–4.

44. Horrigan JP, Barnhill LJ. Risperidone and PTSD in boys. J Neuropsychiatry Clin Neurosci 1999;11:126–7.

45. Cohen JA, Mannarino AP, Deblinger E. Treating trauma and traumatic grief in chil-dren and adolescents: a clinician's guide. New York: Guilford Press; 2006.

46. Cary CE, McMillen JC. The data behind dissemination: a systematic review of trauma-focused cognitive behavioral therapy for use with children and youth. Child Youth Serv Rev 2012;34:748–57.

47. de Arellano MA, Lyman RD, Jobe-Shields L, et al. Trauma-focused cognitive-behavioral therapy for children and adolescents: assessing the evidence. Psychiatr Serv 2014;65:591–602.
48. Silverman WK, Ortiz CD, Viswesvaran C, et al. Evidence-based psychosocial treatments for children and adolescents exposed to traumatic events. J Clin Child Adolesc Psychol 2008;37:156–83.
49. Black PJ, Woodworth M, Tremblay M, et al. A review of trauma-informed treatment for adolescents. Can Psychol 2012;53:192–203.
50. Hanson RF, Jobe-Shields L. Trauma-focused cognitive behavioral therapy (TF-CBT) for children and adolescents. In: Gold S, Cook J, Dalenberg C, editors. APA handbook of trauma psychology, in press.
51. Pollio E, McLean M, Behl LE, et al. Trauma-focused cognitive behavioral therapy. In: Reece RM, Hanson RF, Sargent J, editors. Treatment of child abuse: common ground for mental health, medical, and legal practitioners. 2nd edition. Baltimore (MD): The Johns Hopkins University Press; 2014. p. 31–8.
52. DuMont KA, Widom CS, Czaja SJ. Predictors of resilience in abused and neglected children grown-up: the role of individual and neighborhood characteristics. Child Abuse Negl 2007;31:255–74.
53. Roesler TA, McKenzie N. Effects of childhood trauma on psychological functioning in adults sexually abused as children. J Nerv Ment Dis 1994;182:145–50.
54. Briere JN, Elliot DM. Immediate and long-term impacts of child sexual abuse. Future Child 1994;4:54–69.
55. Felitti VJ, Anda RF. The Adverse Childhood Experiences (ACE) Study. Centers for Disease Control and Prevention; 1997. Available at: http://www.cdc.gov/violenceprevention/acestudy/index.html.
56. Messman-Moore TL, Long PJ. The role of childhood sexual abuse sequelae in the sexual revictimization of women: an empirical review and theoretical reformulation. Clin Psychol Rev 2003;25:537–71.
57. Hornor G. Child maltreatment: screening and anticipatory guidance. J Pediatr Health Care 2013;27:242–50.
58. Flaherty EG, Stirling J. The Committee on Child Abuse and Neglect The pediatrician's role in child maltreatment prevention. Pediatrics 2010;126:833.
59. Leder M, Emans S, Halfler J, et al. Addressing sexual abuse in the primary care setting. Pediatrics 1999;104:270–5.
60. Facts for families: child sexual abuse. American Academy of Child and Adolescent Psychiatry; 2011. Available at: https://www.aacap.org/AACAP/Families_and_Youth/Facts_for_Families/FFF-Guide/Child-Sexual-Abuse-009.aspx. Accessed February 26, 2016.
61. Carole J, Crawford-Jakubiak J. The evaluation of children in the primary care setting when sexual abuse is suspected. Pediatrics 2013;13:103.
62. Child Welfare Information Gateway. Mandatory reporters of child abuse and neglect. Washington, DC: U.S. Department of Health and Human Services, Children's Bureau; 2014.
63. American Psychiatric Association. 2013. Available at: http://www.dsm5.org/Documents/PTSD%20Fact%20Sheet.pdf. Accessed July 6, 2015.
64. Muris P, Merckelbach H, Körver P, et al. Screening for trauma in children and adolescents: the validity of the Traumatic Stress Disorder Scale of the screen for child anxiety related emotional disorders. J Clin Child Psychol 2000;29(3):406–13.

Psychopharmacology in Primary Care Settings

Joseph J. Benich III, MD[a],*, Scott W. Bragg, PharmD[b], John R. Freedy, MD, PhD[c]

KEYWORDS

- Depression • Antidepressants • Anxiety • Anxiolytics • Bipolar • Pharmacotherapy
- Antipsychotics

KEY POINTS

- Second-generation antidepressants are effective treatment options for both major depressive disorder and generalized anxiety disorder, so medication selection should be based on prior response to treatments, dosing frequency, patient preference, medication side effects, comorbid conditions, and cost.
- Adverse effects of medications can be used to control additional or predominant symptoms of the targeted mental disorders, such as insomnia.
- The best indications for benzodiazepines are short-term use for anxiety disorders, acute agitation, and seizure disorders.
- For schizophrenia, start either an atypical or typical antipsychotic and then reassess after an appropriate trial of 3 to 6 months of therapy. Clozapine can be considered after 2 failed courses of first-line neuroleptics.
- Treatment of patients with bipolar disorder may benefit from lamotrigine, carbamazepine, lithium, antidepressants, or antipsychotics. The first-line medications to consider are lamotrigine and lithium.

INTRODUCTION

In the United States, primary care settings (family medicine, general internal medicine, general pediatrics, and office-based obstetrics and gynecology practices) have for decades served as the de facto US mental health services system.[1] Among adults, 18.5% have a mental health problem each year.[2] For children aged 13 to 18 years,

Disclosure: The authors do not have any commercial or financial conflicts of interest or any funding sources to disclose.
[a] Department of Family Medicine, Medical University of South Carolina, 5 Charleston Center, Suite 263, Charleston, SC 29425, USA; [b] Department of Family Medicine, South Carolina College of Pharmacy (MUSC Campus), Medical University of South Carolina, 5 Charleston Center, Suite 263, Charleston, SC 29425, USA; [c] Department of Family Medicine, College of Medicine, Medical University of South Carolina, 5 Charleston Center, Suite 263, Charleston, SC 29425, USA
* Corresponding author.
E-mail address: benichjj@musc.edu

the annual prevalence for any mental disorder is 13.1%.[3] Typically, fewer than half of adults or children with a mental health problem are seen by a professional each year (between one-fourth and one-third is a typical treatment rate for various mental disorders). Among people who do see some type of professional for a mental health issue, more than half of these consultations are provided by primary care providers within primary care settings.[4] Even more remarkable, referrals to specialty mental health services most often result in failure to engage in treatment. When mental health treatment is offered within the primary care setting, 2 desirable things result: (1) the patient is more likely to become engaged with treatment, and (2) both mental health and physical health indicators for internally referred patients engaged in mental health treatment are likely to improve.[5]

Primary care clinicians must consider the provision of high-quality mental health services within the primary care setting as a best-practices standard. Borrowing from the *Crossing the Quality Chasm* report from the Institute on Medicine, patient-centered care requires "providing care that is respectful of and responsive to individual patient preferences, needs, and values, and ensuring that patient values guide all clinical decisions."[6] Patients often prefer to get mental health care from their primary care providers if they are willing to receive care at all for mental health issues. Patients have various motivations for seeking and accepting mental health treatment from their primary care providers. These motives include 1 or more of the following:

1. Accessibility: an appointment with a primary care provider is usually easier to obtain than with a mental health provider.
2. Cost-effectiveness: it generally costs less to see a primary care provider than it does to see a psychiatrist or other mental health provider, and insurance may limit access for mental health services.
3. Privacy: it is common to visit a primary care provider and for a wide variety of reasons, so patients feel reassured by this anonymity because no one knows whether they are being seen for high blood pressure, depression, or some other reason.
4. Effectiveness: mental health treatments offered within primary care settings often reduce symptoms and enhance function as well as quality of life.
5. Relationship/sense of community: a well-managed doctor-patient relationship is a source of support and hope for many primary care patients, and, by extension, a well-trained primary care staff can serve as a reflection of the clinician's empathy for and encouragement of the patient.
6. Integration: improved mental health often improves health habits and physical health as well, so both patients and providers benefit by experiencing the positive synergy that can be associated with receiving mental health treatment within primary care settings.

This article focuses on psychopharmacology for the most commonly seen mental health problems among adults in primary care settings (depressive disorders, anxiety disorders, bipolar disorders, and disorders with psychotic features). The intent is for readers to review and apply this information as part of the so-called tool box for most effectively managing adult mental health problems within a primary care setting. Beyond understanding the evidence base for typically used psychotropic medications for adults, other aspects of the primary care providers' mental health tool box should include an understanding of useful psychotherapeutic options (eg, cognitive behavior therapy), available community resources (eg, private and public mental health clinics, area support groups), development of local collaborative care models where possible (integrating primary care, mental health care, and case management), as well as the aforementioned adoption of a patient-centered attitude with regard to providing mental health services in, or at least closely aligned with, the primary care practice.[7] It is within the practice scope of well-trained primary care clinicians to attend to the mental health needs (including treatment preferences) of their patients.[4]

ANTIDEPRESSANTS

Pharmacotherapy is the most often used treatment of depression, with more than 27 million Americans being treated with antidepressants per year.[8] Antidepressants have been shown to be effective compared with placebo in the primary care setting.[9] Antidepressants are classified into the 2 major categories of first-generation and second-generation medications. First-generation medications such as monoamine oxidase inhibitors (MAOIs) and tricyclic antidepressants (TCAs) are not used as often because of the high frequency of side effects. MAOIs can cause malignant hypertension if combined with sympathomimetic medications or tyramine-containing foods (eg, aged cheeses, cured meats, soy sauce, fava beans). TCAs have a high mortality in cases of overdose and also commonly cause anticholinergic side effects.

The more commonly used second-generation antidepressants are classified into 4 major categories: selective serotonin reuptake inhibitors (SSRIs), serotonin-norepinephrine reuptake inhibitors (SNRIs), serotonin modulators, and atypical antidepressants. Studies have shown similar efficacy in treating depressive symptoms across these medication classes.[10] A meta-analysis comparing SNRIs and SSRIs showed both were similarly effective at achieving remission rates among patients with major depressive disorder.[11] Clinicians can focus on other influences, such as co-morbid conditions, when choosing an initial treatment in an attempt to control as many symptoms as possible with the fewest medications. For example, SNRIs have been shown to be superior to SSRIs in controlling the symptoms of fibromyalgia and neuropathic pain.[12,13] Also, bupropion can help depressed patients who are also trying to quit smoking.

Adverse effects are a potential deterrent to any treatment regimen. More than half of patients experience at least 1 side effect from antidepressant medications.[10] Adverse effects from treatment can include insomnia, weight gain, and sexual dysfunction. Caution needs to be exercised to avoid serotonin syndrome, a condition with dangerous blood pressure increase that can occur if SSRIs are combined with certain medications like MAOIs, tramadol, or linezolid. SNRIs have been shown to have higher rates of side effects compared with the other second-generation antidepressants; most commonly nausea and vomiting.[10] Although such adverse reactions can be a reason for discontinuing a medication, clinicians should try to augment therapy by choosing medications that allow the side effects to help control additional symptoms of the depression. For example, trazodone and mirtazapine can be used to effectively treat patients who have insomnia as a major symptom of their depression (**Tables 1–3**).

The issue of suicidality (thoughts, behaviors, and completed suicide) merits special comment with regard to antidepressant medications. In 2004, the US Food and Drug Administration (FDA) issued a black-box warning with regard to the potential risk for suicidal thoughts and behaviors among young people less than 24 years of age, although there was never evidence of an increased number of completed suicides associated with the use of antidepressant medication. This warning was modified in 2007 to note that depression itself was associated with an increased risk for suicidal thoughts and behaviors. Although causality cannot be certain, several notable

Table 1
Selective serotonin reuptake inhibitor adverse effects

Side Effects	Citalopram	Escitalopram	Fluoxetine	Fluvoxamine[a]	Paroxetine	Sertraline
Sexual dysfunction	++	++	++	++	+++	++
Weight gain	+	+	+	+	++	+
GI toxicity	+	+	+	+	+	++
QTc prolongation	+	+	+	+	+	+
Orthostatic hypotension	+	+	+	+	++	+
Insomnia	+	+	++	+	+	++
Drowsiness	±	±	±	+	+	±

Abbreviations: ±, none to minimal; +, mild; ++, moderate; +++, severe; GI, gastrointestinal; QTc, corrected QT interval.

[a] Only approved to treat obsessive compulsive disorder.

Data from Lexicomp Online. Copyright © 1978-2015 Lexicomp, Inc. All Rights Reserved. Available at: http://www.wolterskluwercdi.com/lexicomp-online/.

epidemiologic trends have occurred since the 2004 FDA black-box warning, including:

1. Reduced rate of depression diagnoses for children and adults seen by primary care providers
2. Reduced rates of antidepressant prescriptions for children and adults written by primary care providers
3. No parallel increase in the use of other depression treatments for children or adults (eg, cognitive behavioral psychotherapy, other medications) by primary care providers[14]

Primary care clinicians have an ethical obligation to appropriately assess for and offer treatment of depression among children and adults seeking care within primary care settings.[15,16] Although suicidality does occur among primary care patients (typically at a rate of 2%–3%), careful clinical assessment and management of depressive symptoms (including suicidality) remain the responsibility of primary care providers.

Table 2
SNRI adverse effects

Side Effects	Desvenlafaxine	Duloxetine	Milnacipran[a]	Venlafaxine
Sexual dysfunction	+++	+++	±	+++
Weight gain	±	±	±	±
GI toxicity	++	++	++	++
QTc prolongation	±	±	±	+
Orthostatic hypotension	±	±	±	±
Insomnia	++	++	±	++
Sedation	+	±	+	+

[a] Approved for the treatment of fibromyalgia.

Data from Lexicomp Online. Copyright © 1978-2015 Lexicomp, Inc. All Rights Reserved. Available at: http://www.wolterskluwercdi.com/lexicomp-online/.

Table 3
Serotonin modulator (trazodone and vilazodone) and atypical agent (bupropion and mirtazapine) adverse effects

Side Effects	Trazodone	Vilazodone	Bupropion	Mirtazapine
Sexual dysfunction	+	++	±	+
Weight gain	+	±	±	+++
GI toxicity	+++	+++	+	±
QTc prolongation	++	±	+	+
Orthostatic hypotension	+++	±	±	±
Insomnia	±	++	++	±
Sedation	+++	±	±	+++

Data from Lexicomp Online. Copyright © 1978-2015 Lexicomp, Inc. All Rights Reserved. Available at: http://www.wolterskluwercdi.com/lexicomp-online/.

An overemphasis on an exceedingly rare, although serious, outcome (completed suicide by a primary care patient) should not deter primary care providers from offering an appropriate range of mental health treatments, including well-chosen and carefully monitored antidepressant medication.[17]

Treatment should factor in variables like patient age, treatment adherence, patient past response to treatments, dosing frequency, potential medication interactions, drug precautions/warnings, medication cost, patient preference, and medication side effect profiles.[18] **Table 4** shows the cost of second-generation antidepressants in addition to their dosage range and frequency of dosing.

Table 4
Cost and dosing of second-generation antidepressants

Medication	Estimated Cost for One Month's Treatment ($)	Dose (mg)	Dosing Frequency
Bupropion	16–65	100–150	TID
Citalopram	4–12	20–40	Daily
Desvenlafaxine	137–313	50–100	Daily
Duloxetine	25–102	60–120	Daily
Escitalopram	11–66	10–20	Daily
Fluoxetine	4–12	20–80	Daily
Fluvoxamine[a]	23–70	50–150	BID
Milnacipran[b]	237–255	12.5–100	BID
Mirtazapine	5–45	15–45	QHS
Paroxetine	4–16	20–50	Daily
Sertraline	9–35	50–200	Daily
Trazodone	4–12	50–200	BID to TID
Venlafaxine	15–63	37.5–125	BID to TID
Vilazodone[c]	200	20–40	Daily

Abbreviations: BID, twice a day; QHS, at bedtime; TID, 3 times a day.
[a] Only approved to treat obsessive compulsive disorder.
[b] Nongeneric and approved for treatment of fibromyalgia.
[c] Nongeneric.
Data from GoodRx. Available at: http://www.goodrx.com. Accessed July 1, 2015.

The acute phase of depression treatment occurs from weeks 6 to 12, during which time clinicians need to decide whether the patient is responding to the selected treatment regimen. Duration of therapy is the point of emphasis after an effective medication has been chosen. The second phase of depression treatment is the continuation phase, which typically lasts 4 to 9 months. Clinicians can stop treatment once the depression symptoms have resolved. Those patients who have had prior episodes of depression should continue a third maintenance phase of pharmacotherapy, which can last 1 or more years.[18] **Fig. 1** shows a visual depiction of these 3 phases. In patients with recurrent or persistent depression (3 or more distinct episodes with moderate to severe symptoms in the absence of antidepressant medication), it is appropriate to offer multiyear maintenance pharmacotherapy with biannual to annual follow-up to assess depressive symptoms, medication side effects, functionality, and quality of life.

BENZODIAZEPINES

Benzodiazepines are used in several conditions, including anxiety disorders, seizure disorder, insomnia, alcohol withdrawal, tremor, and agitation. Their anxiolytic and antiseizure effects are thought to be mediated by activity on gamma-aminobutyric acid receptors, resulting in a spike in inhibitory neurotransmitters in the central nervous system. However, several concerns exist with benzodiazepines, including an increase in mental health disorders, central nervous system depression, and respiratory depression, as well as benzodiazepine withdrawal, dependence, and addiction. The FDA requires special prescribing and handling requirements for benzodiazepines by labeling them as controlled substances because of the significant risk of misuse and abuse. Benzodiazepines should not be used in combination with opioid analgesics if possible because of the risk of added respiratory and central nervous system depression that at least doubles the risk of death from drug overdose.[19]

The most appropriate indications for benzodiazepines are short-term use for anxiety disorders, acute agitation, and seizure disorders. Guideline recommendations prefer using antidepressants and nonpharmacologic interventions like cognitive behavior therapy for anxiety disorders, but experts think benzodiazepines have a clear role in augmenting therapy.[20] This role seems to be short-term scheduled dosing (days up to 3 months depending on clinical circumstances) to provide quicker treatment response in patients with severe generalized anxiety or panic disorder. As-needed use of benzodiazepines is not preferred despite widespread use on an as-needed basis. With the natural course of panic attacks, these events peak in 10 minutes from the onset and resolve within 30 minutes. However, if using

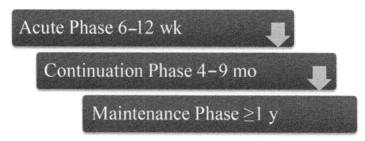

Fig. 1. Treatment algorithm for treating depression to full remission.

oral benzodiazepines, whose onset of action is approximately 30 minutes, they should realistically be dosed regularly, twice or 3 times daily, to have any benefit in reducing panic attacks.[21] A comparison of oral benzodiazepines is given in **Table 5**.

Benzodiazepines are a useful alternative for prompt reversal of seizures when given intravenously, intramuscularly, or rectally. Treatment of severe agitation may warrant intravenous or intramuscular benzodiazepines, but they can also be scheduled orally if the patient is alert and oriented. Benzodiazepines also remain the treatment of choice for severe alcohol withdrawal and prevention of seizures or delirium tremens. However, they should not be routinely used chronically with seizure disorders because of the noted adverse effects and advantages of other anticonvulsants. Similarly, benzodiazepines should be avoided for insomnia because of negative effects on sleep architecture. They may decrease sleep latency and prolong total sleep time, but they seem to impair slow wave sleep (deep-wave sleep), which is thought to be the most restorative stage of sleep.[22] For insomnia, the mainstay of therapy should be sleep hygiene modifications, but the nonbenzodiazepine hypnotics like zolpidem could be an alternative to benzodiazepines because they do not impair slow wave sleep.

NONBENZODIAZEPINE ANXIOLYTICS

SSRIs and SNRIs are also effective options for treating anxiety disorder, with a number needed to treat of 5 to achieve a clinical response in 1 patient.[23] Escitalopram, paroxetine, venlafaxine, and duloxetine are approved by the FDA for use in treating generalized anxiety disorder (GAD). Treatment is typically started at a low dose and slowly titrated up until symptoms are controlled with the lowest effective dose possible in an attempt to minimize side effects. After 4 or more weeks of treatment, the patient is evaluated for response to titrate up the dose or to change medications because of inefficacy. The same influencing factors as those used to choose a medication to treat depression are considered when selecting an anxiety medication.

Tricyclic antidepressants, such as imipramine, have been shown to effectively treat GAD.[23] However, severe side effects like cardiotoxicity and the availability of better-tolerated treatment options makes this a second-tier option.

Buspirone is a 5-hydroxytryptamine agonist and is FDA approved for the treatment of anxiety. Doses are started at 7.5 mg twice a day and titrated up 5 mg per day every 3 days until a therapeutic dose of 20 to 30 mg twice a day to 3 times a day is achieved, with a maximum dose of 60 mg per day. Trials have shown it to be effective at treating

Table 5 Benzodiazepine comparison for oral preparations				
Drug	Usual Dose (mg)	Peak Onset (h)	Half-life[a] (h)	Duration
Clonazepam	0.25–1	1–4	17–60	Intermediate
Diazepam	2–10	0.25–2.5	44–100	Long
Lorazepam	1–2	~2	~12	Intermediate
Oxazepam	10–15	~3	6–11	Intermediate

[a] Half-life listed considers parent drug and active metabolites.

Data from Lexicomp Online. Copyright © 1978-2015 Lexicomp, Inc. All Rights Reserved. Available at: http://www.wolterskluwercdi.com/lexicomp-online/.

anxiety and well tolerated, especially in the elderly, but not superior to SSRI or SNRI options.[24,25] Buspirone is more often used to augment SSRI or SNRI therapy for GAD.

A Cochrane Review showed that hydroxyzine is more effective than placebo for treating GAD (odds ratio [OR], 0.30; 95% confidence interval [CI], 0.15–0.58) and is well tolerated (OR, 1.49; 95% CI, 0.92–2.40).[26] Hydroxyzine was equivalent in terms of efficacy, acceptability and tolerability compared with buspirone and chlordiaz-epoxide, although it had a significant increase in sedation compared with other therapies.[26]

NEUROLEPTICS

In recent years, antipsychotics, also known as neuroleptics, have been approved and prescribed for several psychiatric illnesses. The first typical antipsychotic chlorprom-azine was approved in the 1950s for schizophrenia, but now indications for newer atypical antipsychotics include major depression, bipolar depression, acute agitation, Tourette syndrome, and irritability associated with autism.[27] They also are used off la-bel for insomnia, nausea or vomiting, posttraumatic stress disorder, delirium, and irri-tability with dementia.[28] The older class of neuroleptics, termed typical antipsychotics (eg, chlorpromazine, haloperidol), primarily work through dopamine D_2 receptor blockade to treat the positive symptoms of schizophrenia, including hallucinations, delusions, thought disorders, and movement disorders. Newer generations of neuro-leptics, termed atypical antipsychotics (eg, aripiprazole, lurasidone, olanzapine, que-tiapine), work on dopamine D_2 receptor blockade but also affect other dopamine receptors, serotonin, glutamate, alpha$_1$-adrenergic receptors, and histamine H_1 re-ceptors. These widespread effects are thought to treat some of the negative symp-toms of schizophrenia, including flat affect, anhedonia, inattention, impaired memory, and poor executive function. They may also help in other psychiatric illnesses like major depression and bipolar depression that might be caused in part by imbal-ances in several of these neurotransmitters.

However, many clinicians are concerned with overuse of these neuroleptics, because of their significant side effect profile and early use in so many psychiatric and neurologic conditions.[29] Some of the most severe adverse side effects include neuroleptic malig-nant syndrome, extrapyramidal reactions, cardiac arrhythmias, blood dyscrasias, metabolic disease, cardiovascular events, and death. In 2008, the FDA released major cautions on antipsychotics with a black-box warning when used in patients with dementia-related psychosis because of a 60% to 70% increase in mortality.[30,31] Other concerns with antipsychotics were published by the American Psychiatric Association in 2013 as part of the Choosing Wisely campaign, warning physicians and patients about potential inappropriate use that was becoming common with this medication class. These warnings include not prescribing neuroleptics without appropriate moni-toring, not routinely prescribing 2 or more antipsychotics, not using antipsychotics as first line in children without a psychotic disorder, and not using neuroleptics for insomnia.[32] As a result of these concerns, judicious use of neuroleptics is warranted.

With such potential for adverse patient outcomes and signs of significant overuse,[33] prescribers must ask the question, "Who is an appropriate candidate to use an anti-psychotic?" Moreover, it might also be asked, "How are antipsychotics monitored to minimize the potential for adverse effects?" To help identify appropriate candidates for antipsychotics in primary care, **Table 6** shows the appropriateness based on the indication for the antipsychotic.

These general classifications are based on guidelines from the Choosing Wisely campaign and in reviewing treatment algorithms for each disease state. Monitoring

Table 6
Antipsychotic appropriateness per indication

Appropriateness	Indication
Appropriate	• Schizophrenia/schizoaffective disorder • Hallucinations/delusions • Severe bipolar
Potentially appropriate	• Mild bipolar • Delirium
Potentially inappropriate	• Behavioral symptoms with dementia • Children or adolescents for any indication except psychotic disorders • Depression or anxiety
Inappropriate	• Insomnia • Posttraumatic stress syndrome • Intractable nausea and vomiting

Data from Refs.[20,30,32,37,40]

for antipsychotic side effects is also important considering the number of problems that can arise, as previously mentioned. The recommended monitoring tests are summarized in **Table 7**.

Choice of treatment with antipsychotics should be based on the patient's past response, patient preference, treatment adherence, medication side effects, drug precautions/warnings, and cost. Mixed evidence exists on the superiority of atypical antipsychotics compared with typical antipsychotics with regard to effectiveness, discontinuation rate, and rate of adverse effects.[34–36] The most effective antipsychotic is thought to be clozapine, but it is typically reserved to third or fourth line based on the

Table 7
Recommended neuroleptic monitoring tests

Test	Baseline	Weekly	Monthly	Every 3 mo	Every 6 mo	Annually
Personal and family history	x	—	—	—	—	x
Fasting glucose	x	—	—	x	—	x
Blood pressure	x	—	—	x	—	x
Fasting lipid profile	x	—	—	x	—	x
CBC	x	x[a]	x[a]	—	—	—
Liver and renal function	x	—	—	—	x	x
Thyroid[b]	x	—	—	—	x	x
Eye examination	x	—	—	—	—	x
Abnormal involuntary movement scale	x	x[c]	—	—	x	—

Abbreviation: CBC, complete blood count.
  [a] Clozapine absolute neutrophil count (ANC)/white blood cell count weekly for 6 months, then every other week for 6 months, then monthly; monitor other agents weekly to monthly if having a low ANC.
  [b] Only quetiapine.
  [c] Weekly until on a stable dose for greater than 2 weeks.
  Data from Lexicomp Online. Copyright © 1978-2015 Lexicomp, Inc. All Rights Reserved. Available at: http://www.wolterskluwercdi.com/lexicomp-online/.

rare life-threatening side effect, agranulocytosis.[37] The prescribing of clozapine is restricted to physicians (typically psychiatrists) and pharmacists who participate in the clozapine patient registry.[38] Several generic options exist, including all atypical antipsychotics, clozapine, quetiapine, olanzapine, and risperidone. When considering side effect profiles, refer to **Table 8** to determine general medication tolerability.[39]

In practice, start either an atypical or typical antipsychotic based on the previously discussed factors and then reassess after an appropriate trial of 3 to 6 months of therapy. If the patient fails 1 course, consider an alternative agent; if the patient fails 2 courses, it is reasonable to consider clozapine with appropriate monitoring. As a general rule, only use 2 antipsychotics concomitantly if the plan is to stop one and start the other with dosage reduction and titration respectively.[32]

BIPOLAR DISORDER MEDICATIONS

Bipolar disorder is classified into bipolar I, bipolar II, and rapid cycling disease. Pharmacotherapy to target each is slightly different, but classically drugs with mood-stabilizing properties have been used. The term mood stabilizers may not be the best term, because there are no specific definitions or single class of drugs that provide mood stabilization. Rather, clinicians should look for agents with antimanic properties and medications targeted for bipolar depression if needed as an adjunct.[40]

Patients with bipolar I have episodes of mania and depression, whereas patients with bipolar II have primarily depressive episodes with occasional hypomania. Rapid cycling bipolar is defined as having 4 or more episodes of depression, mania, or hypomania in a 12-month period. These patients may transition to times of full remission for several months between episodes or switch directly from mania to depression or vice versa. Patients with severe mania may warrant earlier treatment with an antipsychotic in combination with lithium or valproate compared with patients with less severe mania. Short-term use of benzodiazepines may also be appropriate if patients present with significant agitation. However, if a patient has hypomania then monotherapy with lithium or valproate may be the most appropriate option, particularly if the patient has used either of these medications with good response in the past.[40]

Side Effects	Typical Agents	Clozapine	Risperidone	Olanzapine	Quetiapine	Aripiprazole
Sedation	± to +++	+++	±	++	++	±
Weight gain	± to ++	+++	+	+++	++	±
Diabetes	± to +	+++	+	+++	++	±
QTc prolongation	+	++	+	+	+	±
Orthostatic hypotension	± to +++	+++	++	+	++	±
Prolactin	+++	±	+++	±	±	±
EPS	+ to +++	±	± to +++	± to +	±	± to +
TD	+++	±	± to ++	±	±	±

Table 8
Antipsychotic adverse effects

Abbreviations: EPS, extrapyramidal symptoms; TD, tardive dyskinesia.
Data from Glick ID, He X, Davis JM. First-generation antipsychotics: current status. Prim Psychiatr 2006;13(12):51–8.

To make a determination on the best initial medication for mania or hypomania, take a detailed patient history, consider the current clinical presentation, identify patient expectations, and think about long-term side effects with each alternative. Examples of medication options that likely should be cautioned or avoided based on a patients' history are both lithium and valproate in pregnant patients because both drugs cause potential fetal harm. Also, **Table 9** shows the monitoring parameters on lithium and valproate.

If a patient is started on an antipsychotic medication be mindful of the needed monitoring parameters and potential adverse effects previously mentioned (see **Tables 7 and 8**). In addition, when assessing patient response and a partial response is seen, consider increasing the current dose of the antimanic agent and/or augment with one of the other agents.

Treatment of patients with bipolar depression may benefit from lamotrigine, carbamazepine, lithium, antidepressants, or antipsychotics. The first-line medications to consider are lamotrigine and lithium. Both medications have a slower onset of action and require monitoring levels with lithium or slow dose titration with lamotrigine. The big concern with rapid dose titration on lamotrigine is a life-threatening skin reaction such as Stevens-Johnson syndrome; therefore, the dose is slowly increased weekly to goal dosages between 200 and 400 mg daily. Carbamazepine and antidepressants are good second-line alternatives. Conflicting evidence exists about the potential for a switch to a manic or hypomanic state after starting an antidepressant.[41,42] It is generally recommended to not use an antidepressant alone to prevent this switch phenomenon. Use of antidepressants in combination with antimanic medications has not shown any increased risk of a manic switch.[42] Clinicians typically reserve use of

Table 9
Recommended bipolar medications monitoring tests

Test	Baseline	Twice Weekly	Monthly	Every 3 mo	Every 6 mo	Annually
Lithium						
Lithium level	—	x[a]	—	x	x	—
Renal function	x	—	—	x	—	x
Electrolytes	x	—	—	x	—	x
TSH	x	—	—	x	—	x
Pregnancy hCG	x	—	—	—	—	—
ECG	x[b]	—	—	—	—	—
CBC	x	—	—	—	—	x
Valproate						
Valproate level	—	x[c]	—	—	x	x
Liver enzymes	x	—	x	—	x	x
CBC	x	—	x	—	x	x

Abbreviations: ECG, electrocardiogram; hCG, human chorionic gonadotropin; TSH, thyroid-stimulating hormone.
[a] Acute mania goal: 0.5 to 1.2 mEq/L and maintenance goal: 0.6 to 1 mEq/L.
[b] Only for patients more than 40 years old; repeat only as needed.
[c] Acute mania goal: 50 to 125 µg/mL; maintenance goal debatable-some advocate for 75 to 100 µg/mL.
Courtesy of Lexicomp, Inc, 1978-2015. Available at: http://www.wolterskluwercdi.com/lexicomp-online/.

antipsychotics for patients with depression with psychotic features or those failing other depression treatment options.[40]

SUMMARY

Axis I psychiatric conditions are prevalent in the primary care population. Depression, anxiety, bipolar, and conditions with psychotic features are only some of the mental disorders commonly treated by primary care physicians. Psychopharmacology requires controlling a patient's predominant symptoms while taking into consideration patient age, treatment compliance, past response to treatments, dosing frequency, patient preference, medication side effects, potential medication interactions, drug precautions/warnings, and cost. Second-generation antidepressants are the favored therapy to treat major depressive disorder. Targeting comorbid conditions and effectively using medication adverse events to control additional symptoms are effective strategies. In the short term, benzodiazepines are properly used to control anxiety disorders, acute agitation, and seizure disorders. Atypical or typical antipsychotics are used to control the symptoms associated with schizophrenia. Clozapine can be considered if 2 other courses of medication have failed 3-month to 6-month trials. Treatment of patients with bipolar disorder may benefit from lamotrigine, carbamazepine, lithium, antidepressants, or antipsychotics. First-line medications to consider are lamotrigine and lithium. The goal of psychopharmacotherapy is to minimize or eliminate symptoms and to return patients to their maximal level of functioning.

REFERENCES

1. Reiger DA, Goldberg ID, Taube CA. The de facto U.S. mental health services system: a public health perspective. Arch Gen Psychiatry 1978;35(6):685–93.
2. National Institute of Mental Health. Any disorder among adults. Available at: http://www.nimh.nih.gov/health/statistics/prevalence/any-disorder-among-adults.shtml. Accessed August 5, 2015.
3. National Institute of Mental Health. Any disorder among children. Available at: http://www.nimh.nih.gov/health/statistics/prevalence/any-disorder-among-children.shtml. Accessed August 5, 2015.
4. Miller BF, Druss B. The role of family physicians in mental health care delivery in the United States: implications for health reform. J Am Board Fam Med 2013; 26(2):111–3.
5. Kessler R. Mental health care treatment initiation when mental health services are incorporated into primary care practice. J Am Board Fam Med 2012;25(2):255–9.
6. Institute of Medicine. Crossing the quality chasm: a new health system for the 21st century. Washington, DC: National Academy Press; 2001.
7. Thota AB, Sipe TA, Byard GJ, et al. Collaborative care to improve the management of depressive disorders: a community guide systematic review and meta-analysis. Am J Prev Med 2012;42(5):525–38.
8. Olfson M, Marcus SC. National patterns in antidepressant medication treatment. Arch Gen Psychiatry 2009;66(8):848–56.
9. Arroll B, Elley CR, Fishman T, et al. Antidepressants versus placebo for depression in primary care. Cochrane Database Syst Rev 2009;(3):CD007954.
10. Gartlehner G, Hansen RA, Morgan LC, et al. Comparative benefits and harms of second-generation antidepressants for treating major depressive disorder: an updated meta-analysis. Ann Intern Med 2011;155(11):772–85.

11. Machado M, Einarson TR. Comparison of SSRIs and SNRIs in major depressive disorder: a meta-analysis of head-to-head randomized clinical trials. J Clin Pharm Ther 2010;35(2):177–88.
12. Saarto T, Wiffen PJ. Antidepressants for neuropathic pain. Cochrane Database Syst Rev 2007;(4):CD005454.
13. Hauser W, Urrutia G, Tort S, et al. Serotonin and norepinephrine reuptake inhibitors for fibromyalgia syndrome. Cochrane Database Syst Rev 2013;(1):CD010292.
14. Friedman RA. Antidepressants' black box warning-10 years later. N Engl J Med 2014;371(18):1666–8.
15. Colonge N, Petitti DB, DeWitt TG. Screening for depression in adults. U.S. Preventative Services Task Force recommendation statement. Ann Intern Med 2009;151(11):784–92.
16. Colonge N, Petitti DB, DeWitt TG. Screening and treatment for major depressive disorder in children and adolescents: U.S. Preventative Services Task Force recommendation statement. Pediatrics 2009;123(4):1223–8.
17. O'Connor E, Gaynes B, Burda BU, et al. Screening for suicide risk in primary care: a systematic evidence review for the U.S. Preventative Services Task Force. Rockville (MD): Agency for Healthcare Research and Quality; 2013.
18. Qaseem A, Snow V, Denberg TD, et al. Using second-generation antidepressants to treat depressive disorders: a clinical practice guideline from the American College of Physicians. Ann Intern Med 2008;149(10):725–33.
19. Park TW, Saitz R, Ganoczy D, et al. Benzodiazepine prescribing patterns and deaths from drug overdose among US veterans receiving opioid analgesics: case-cohort study. BMJ 2015;350:h2698.
20. Bandelow B, Sher L, Bunevicius R, et al. Guidelines for the pharmacological treatment of anxiety disorders, obsessive-compulsive disorder and posttraumatic stress disorder in primary care. Int J Psychiatry Clin Pract 2012;16:77–84.
21. Lexicomp Online®. Pediatric & neonatal Lexi-Drugs®. Hudson (OH): LexiComp; 2015.
22. Proctor A, Bianchi MT. Clinical pharmacology in sleep medicine. ISRN Pharmacol 2012;2012:914168.
23. Kapczinski F, Lima M, Souza JS, et al. Antidepressants for generalized anxiety disorder. Cochrane Database Syst Rev 2003;(2):CD003592.
24. Davidson JR, Dupont RL, Hedges D, et al. Efficacy, safety, and tolerability of venlafaxine extended release and buspirone in outpatients with generalized anxiety disorder. J Clin Psychiatry 1999;60(8):528–35.
25. Mokhber N, Azarpazhooh MR, Khajehdaluee M, et al. Randomized, single-blind, trial of sertraline and buspirone for treatment of elderly patients with generalized anxiety disorder. Psychiatry Clin Neurosci 2010;64(2):128–33.
26. Guaiana G, Barbui C, Cipriani A. Hydroxyzine for generalized anxiety disorder. Cochrane Database Syst Rev 2010;(12):CD006815.
27. Otsuka America Pharmaceutical, Inc. Abilify® (aripiprazole) tablets prescribing information. Rockville (MD): 2005.
28. Eli Lilly and Company. Zyprexa® (olanzapine) tablets. Indianapolis (IN): 2005.
29. Iritani KM, et al. Antipsychotic drug use: HHS has initiatives to reduce use among older adults in nursing homes, but should expand efforts to other settings. GAO-15-211. 2015.
30. Gill SS, Bronskill SE, Normand SL, et al. Antipsychotic drug use and mortality in older adults with dementia. Ann Intern Med 2007;146:775–86.

31. Schneeweiss S, Setoguchi S, Brookhart A, et al. Risk of death associated with the use of conventional versus atypical antipsychotic drugs among elderly patients. CMAJ 2007;176:627–32.

32. American Psychiatric Association. Five things physicians and patients should question. Choosing Wisely ABIM Foundation; 2015.

33. Brown T. 100 best-selling, most prescribed branded drugs through march. Medscape Medical News; 2015. WebMD, LLC.

34. Leucht S, Barnes TRE, Kissling W, et al. Relapse prevention in schizophrenia with new-generation antipsychotics: a systematic review and exploratory meta-analysis of randomized, controlled trials. Am J Psychiatry 2003;160:1209–22.

35. Lieberman JA, Stroup TS, McEvoy JP, et al. Effectiveness of antipsychotic drugs in patients with chronic schizophrenia. N Engl J Med 2005;353:1209–23.

36. Jones PB, Barnes TRE, Davies L, et al. Randomized controlled trial of the effect on quality of life of second vs first generation antipsychotic drugs in schizophrenia. Arch Gen Psychiatry 2006;63:1079–87.

37. Chakos M, Lieberman J, Hoffman E, et al. Effectiveness of second-generation antipsychotics in patients with treatment-resistant schizophrenia: a review and meta-analysis of randomized trials. Am J Psychiatry 2001;158(4):518–26.

38. Teva Clozapine Patient Registry. Available at: http://www.clozapineregistry.com. Accessed August 5, 2015.

39. Glick ID, He X, Davis JM. First-generation antipsychotics: current status. Prim Psychiatr 2006;13(12):51–8.

40. Bipolar disorder: the management of bipolar in adults, children and adolescents, in primary and secondary care. National Collaborating Centre for Mental Health (UK); 2006. p. 1–76.

41. Sachs GS, Nierenberg AA, Calabrese JR, et al. Effectiveness of adjunctive antidepressant treatment for bipolar depression. N Engl J Med 2007;356:1711–22.

42. Viktorin A, Lichtenstein P, Thase ME, et al. The risk of switch to mania in patients with bipolar disorder during treatment with an antidepressant alone and in combination with a mood stabilizer. Am J Psychiatry 2014;171:1067–73.

Psychiatric Emergencies

Santina Wheat, MD, MPH*, Dorothy Dschida, MD,
Mary R. Talen, PhD

KEYWORDS

• Suicide • Homicide • Mania • Psychosis • Agitation • Psychiatric emergency

KEY POINTS

• Psychiatric emergencies, such as mania, psychosis, and suicidal or homicidal ideation, present as an acute disturbance of thought, behavior, or mood that require prompt intervention to prevent imminent danger.
• The first priority in a psychiatric emergency is ensuring the safety of the patient and those surrounding.
• Initial assessment should consist of a thorough history and physical examination, to rule out underlying medical causes, while simultaneously establishing a safe environment for patient and clinician.
• It is imperative to debrief with the patient, family, and the health care team following the treatment of a psychiatric emergency.
• There are important legal considerations, particularly concerning involuntary admission, surrounding psychiatric emergencies.

INTRODUCTION

A psychiatric emergency is defined by the American Psychiatric Association as "an acute disturbance in thought, behavior, mood, or social relationship, which requires immediate intervention as defined by the patient, family, or social unit." Such emergencies require immediate intervention to save the patient and/or others from imminent danger. Patients who present with a psychiatric emergency typically have a diagnosis of mania, acute psychosis, suicidal ideation, or homicidal ideation. The causes of these extreme disturbances in patients' behaviors can be multifaceted and caused by substance use, medical illness, mood disorder, or extreme anxiety and trauma. Ninety percent of patients who have been suicidal also have a psychiatric diagnosis, such as major depression, substance abuse, or schizophrenia. It is also estimated that up to 50% of patients with psychiatric emergencies have a coexisting medical disease. Thus, medical screening is important in identifying physical conditions that may be the cause of, or contributing factors to, the psychiatric emergency.[1]

Northwestern McGaw Family Medicine Residency Program, Erie Family Heath Center, 2750 West North Avenue, Chicago, IL 60647, USA
* Corresponding author.
E-mail address: swheat@eriefamilyhealth.org

Prim Care Clin Office Pract 43 (2016) 341–354
http://dx.doi.org/10.1016/j.pop.2016.01.009   **primarycare.theclinics.com**

Psychiatric emergencies are frequent in hospital and outpatient settings. The reported percentage of emergency department visits that are psychiatric emergencies varies from 6% to 25%.[1,2] Additionally, 10% of primary care visits are for psychiatric emergencies.[2] More importantly, medical providers are the front line in assessing patients who are at risk for suicide. However, primary care providers have not adequately detected the level of risk of patients with suicidal thoughts and behaviors.[3] Although suicidal ideation is present in 2% to 7% of all primary care patients, primary care providers have low rates of inquiry, detection, and intervention.[4–8] It is estimated that 50% of patients who committed suicide had been seen by their primary care physician within 1 month of their death,[1,4] and 20% of adults who die by suicide visited their primary care physician within 24 hours of their death.[9] Consequently, medical providers, including nursing and support staff, need to be trained in the assessment, treatment, and management of these patients.

SCREENING/DIAGNOSIS: PSYCHIATRIC AND MEDICAL ASSESSMENTS

The most important first step in the management of a psychiatric emergency is the initial evaluation. An evaluation should take place in a quiet, private room where the safety of the patient, provider, staff, and other individuals can be maintained. Whenever there is a patient who is extremely agitated, aggressive, or suicidal, the health care team needs to be aware and alert. Patients who need a crisis intervention in a psychiatric emergency typically fall into three main categories: (1) acute psychosis and mania, (2) suicidal and depressed patients, and (3) aggressive and homicidal patients. For each type of psychiatric crisis, the screening and management process may differ and require specific types of interventions.

Acute Psychosis and Mania

Patients with acute psychosis and manic behaviors present with eccentric and exaggerated behaviors; unusual, disorganized, and paranoid thinking; and intense or inappropriate emotional expressions. It is particularly important in the initial evaluation of patients with mania and acute psychosis to screen for organic diseases that may be causing these symptoms. These medical conditions may include delirium, infections, metabolic/endocrine disorders, medications, substance abuse/withdrawal, and central nervous system disorders (**Table 1**).[1] This step is crucial to ensure correct diagnosis and to exclude toxic substances or a medical disorder as the cause.[10,11]

Assessing the past medical history of the patient may assist in the detection of a physical condition versus a purely psychiatric disorder (**Boxes 1** and **2**).[1] If the mania or psychosis is caused by a medical condition, the treatment is different. For example, delirium is an acute state of confusion or disturbance of consciousness caused by a medical illness, and this diagnosis changes the goals and medical management. The four key elements that distinguish delirium from acute psychosis include (1) time course, (2) disturbance of consciousness, (3) change of cognition, and (4) evidence of medical cause.[1]

After safety is established for patient and staff, the next step of the evaluation is to obtain a history of the incident; ask for a description of what happened during a crisis event. This information should be obtained from the patient; family; friends; or even individuals who observed the patient, such as bystanders, police, or neighbors. Providers should also review prior hospital records, if possible.[1,4,10,11] Obtaining information from family members and others involved in the life of the patient is particularly important, especially when the patient is cognitively impaired, agitated, paranoid, or having difficulty contributing to the history for other reasons.[4]

Table 1
Differential diagnosis for patients with mania or acute psychosis

Infections	Bacterial and viral meningitis	Herpes simplex encephalitis	Symptomatic infections (urinary tract infections, Pneumonia)
Metabolic derangements/ endocrine abnormalities	Hypothyroid Hyperthyroid	Diabetes mellitus • Hyperglycemia • Hypoglycemia	—
Medications	Polypharmacy	Anticholinergic agents	—
Substance abuse and withdrawal	—	—	—
Central nervous system disorders	Epilepsy	—	—

Data from Sood TR, McStay CM. Evaluation of the psychiatric patient. Emerg Med Clin North Am 2009;27(4):669–83, ix; and Hirschfeld RM, Russell JM. Assessment and treatment of suicidal patients. N Engl J Med 1997;337(13):910–5.

After obtaining the history, the clinician should determine how alert and oriented the patient is to person, place, and situation. The clinician can then assess for dissociation from reality. This may include assessing for hallucinations and delusions, listening for disorganized thinking or behavior, tangential speech, and observing for blunted affect and avolition. This includes assessing activities of daily living, such as hygiene or eating, and instrumental activities of daily living, such as shopping or managing money. Next, the clinician should obtain the past medical history including psychiatric history and history of substance use. The physical examination should include vital signs, general appearance, attention, and interaction. A full neurologic examination including assessment of alertness, orientation, strength, sensation, cranial nerves, gait, cerebellar tests, and reflexes should be done. Finally, specific organ systems should be assessed particularly looking for signs of infection, hepatic dysfunction, trauma, and cardiac disease.[1] Provisional diagnoses of the mental disorder and any potentially contributing medical diagnoses or substance use should be made to guide further evaluation and management decisions (**Fig. 1**).[4]

Screening tools can be useful for assessment of the patient with acute psychosis or mania. The Mini Mental Status Exam and the Quick Confusion Scale are useful tools to help providers evaluate a patient's cognitive functioning.[12] In addition, a patient's level of agitation is assessed using the Agitation Behavior Scale or the Behavioral Activity

Box 1
Patients likely to have coexisting medical illness

1. Elderly

2. History of substance abuse

3. No history of psychiatric history

4. Pre-existing medical illness

5. Lower socioeconomic status

Data from Sood TR, McStay CM. Evaluation of the psychiatric patient. Emerg Med Clin North Am 2009;27(4):669–83, ix.

Box 2
Key points of assessment of suicidal patient

- History
- Current circumstances
- Mental state
- Suicidal thinking
- Suicidal behaviors

Data from Practice guideline for the assessment and treatment of patients with suicidal behaviors. Am J Psychiatry 2003;160(11 Suppl):1–60.

Ratings Scale.[1,13] Failure to refer to standardized criteria for assessing the level of risk is a common pitfall and can lead to inadequately triaging the patient.[14]

After a history and examination have been completed, the clinician may consider laboratory studies. If a patient has a significant psychiatric history, laboratory studies are unlikely to add much useful information. However, certain tests can be done to rule out common medical causes and substance use. The diagnostic evaluation should be dictated by the specific psychiatric symptoms and the patient's history and physical examination.[15] For example, a urine drug screen or blood alcohol level may be useful in assessing for intoxication and specific substance abuse. A lumbar puncture is only useful in the setting of suspected meningitis or encephalitis. Computed tomography scan or other imaging is unlikely to add much information if there are no focal findings on examination, except in the case of an elderly patient.[1,16]

Suicidal and Homicidal Ideation

The evaluation of a patient with suicidal ideation is different than that of a patient with acute psychosis or mania. This evaluation is done to identify factors that increase or decrease risk of suicide, to address immediate safety to determine the most appropriate setting for treatment, and to develop a differential diagnosis that can further guide the plan of treatment. Throughout this evaluation, it is important for the clinician to elicit details surrounding the patient's history and situation, and to maintain a good rapport with the patient while demonstrating empathy.[4]

Similar to the assessment of patients with other psychiatric emergencies, the clinician should identify specific psychiatric signs and symptoms and assess for immediate safety (**Box 3**). During questioning of the patient, the clinician should inquire about past suicidal behavior and frequency of attempts and means. The clinician should also assess for the consumption of drugs and alcohol, because these may make the patient more impulsive, aggressive, and cognitively impaired. There should be an assessment of what treatments the patient has had previously and their response to interventions. An assessment of family history of mental illness and particularly of suicides of family members is important in determining risk. The clinician should determine the current social situation and any recent losses of relationships, status, or employment. The patient should also be evaluated for positive coping skills,

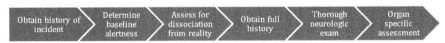

Fig. 1. Evaluation of patient with psychiatric emergency. (*Data from* Sood TR, McStay CM. Evaluation of the psychiatric patient. Emerg Med Clin North Am 2009;27(4):669–83, ix.)

Box 3
Risk factors for eventual suicide

- Male sex
- Age greater than 60
- Widowed or divorced
- White or Native American
- Lives alone
- Unemployed/financial problems
- Recent adverse event
- Depression
- Schizophrenia
- Substance abuse
- History of suicide attempts or ideation
- Feelings of hopelessness
- Panic attacks
- Severe anxiety
- Severe anhedonia

Data from Sood TR, McStay CM. Evaluation of the psychiatric patient. Emerg Med Clin North Am 2009;27(4):669–83, ix; and Hirschfeld RM, Russell JM. Assessment and treatment of suicidal patients. N Engl J Med 1997;337(13):910–5.

---

low self-esteem, cognitions (pessimistic thoughts or "all or nothing" thinking), and dependent psychological needs that may increase or decrease suicide risk.

Ultimately, the clinician must specifically inquire about the patient's intensity of suicidal thoughts, lethality of suicidal plans, accessibility of the means to kill oneself, and current suicidal attempts. Despite clinicians' fears, they will not plant the idea of suicide if they ask about the patient wanting to die or feeling suicidal. It may actually provide a relief to the patient by opening an opportunity for discussion. The patient's specific plan should also be assessed. The patient's belief of the lethality of the plan may be as important as the actual lethality of the plan.[4]

It is important to identify factors that increase a patient's risk for attempting suicide. Some patient factors that generally increase or decrease risk for suicide are not modifiable, but some are and can potentially serve as points of focus for intervention in the short and long term. Scales have been developed to assess suicide risk. Unfortunately, they have high false-positive and false-negative rates, and therefore are not useful for prediction of who is at imminent risk. They can, however, be useful to assist in communication with a patient with suicidal ideation.[4] Other screening tools, such as those for depression and anxiety, can also be useful in helping to develop a treatment plan, although these are not adequate to identify whether the patient is an immediate risk for attempting suicide.[1]

The assessment of the homicidal patient is similar to that of the suicidal patient. Epidemiologic data are not available to determine who is likely to commit homicide. The most reliable predictive risk factor a clinician should assess for is a history of violence and access to weapons. While assessing a patient with homicidal ideation, it is important for the personal safety of the provider to have a quick exit route that cannot be blocked by the patient.[4]

MANAGEMENT GOALS

Once the evaluation has been completed, the clinician must determine whether the patient is willing to form an alliance that allows for successful assessment and treatment. The clinician should determine if the patient is at risk of harm to self or others and then if involuntary treatment and admissions are necessary. The clinician should then develop a specific plan, which includes immediate treatment, disposition, and follow-up.[4]

Acute Psychosis, Mania, and Agitated or Homicidal Patients

The first priorities regardless of the cause of behavior are stabilizing and ensuring the safety of the patient, staff, and family or friends. After ensuring the safety of the patient and staff, the initial approach to an acutely agitated patient should involve assisting the patient to manage his or her stress. The methods of assisting the patient are via behavioral interventions, pharmacologic interventions, or both if necessary.[2,17,18] When the patient has a comorbid medical illness contributing to the psychiatric emergency, it is crucial for the clinician to also treat the medical illness. In some cases, the medical illness is the cause of the psychiatric emergency and is therefore important for the clinician to distinguish. The clinician must distinguish whether these emergencies are secondary to substance or medication use or organic disease using certain clinical criteria, including (1) greater than 30 years with no personal history of psychiatric illness, (2) history of illness or substance use, (3) sudden onset or fluctuation of psychiatric symptoms, (4) confusion and disorientation to time and place, (5) symptoms not corresponding to a specific psychiatric diagnosis, (6) abnormal vital signs, (7) coexisting signs of specific organic illness, and (8) poor response to treatment.[11] The presence of these clinical criteria alters the goals of care. Additionally, the provider must determine the most appropriate location of care. The locations chosen must allow the patient to be treated and have the least amount of restrictiveness while still maintaining safety (**Box 4**).

Suicidal Ideation

Treatment of the patient with suicidal ideation should focus on mitigating risk and strengthening protective factors that are modifiable (**Box 5**). Such modifiable factors include patient safety, associated psychological or social stressors, social support networks, and potentially treatable psychiatric disorders. When managing a patient with suicidal ideation, the clinician must first foster a therapeutic alliance while attending to patient safety. With use of the information gathered in the assessment, a treatment setting should be determined and a treatment plan developed. The clinician should promote adherence to the treatment plan with the patient and any persons providing social support through education and should coordinate care and

---

Box 4
Criteria for psychiatric admission

1. There must be evidence of severe psychiatric illness

2. There must be a clinically indicated evaluation of any suspected medical illness

3. Any medical problems must be sufficiently stable to allow safe transport to and treatment at the state-operated psychiatric facility.

Adapted from Zun LS. Evidence-based evaluation of psychiatric patients. J Emerg Med 2005;28(1):35–9.

Box 5
Suicide treatment plan based on risk

Low Risk: Urgent

- Involve team and social support
- Medication: selective serotonin reuptake inhibitor, sleeping aid
- Close follow-up and community resources
- Remove medications, firearms, knives, and so forth

Moderate Risk: Crisis

- Safety plan: "watch"
- Intensive outpatient treatment
- Medication: selective serotonin reuptake inhibitor, sleeping aid
- Remove harm

High Risk: Emergency

- Inpatient treatment
- Petition for involuntary admission

Data from Practice guideline for the assessment and treatment of patients with suicidal behaviors. Am J Psychiatry 2003;160(11 Suppl):1–60.

---

collaborate with other clinicians as necessary. After establishing and beginning the treatment plan, the patient should be continuously monitored for psychiatric status and treatment response while also reassessing safety and suicide risk.[4,19]

NONPHARMACOLOGIC STRATEGIES
Acute Psychosis, Mania, and Agitated or Homicidal

When approaching a patient with acute agitation, behavioral strategies should be first line. Behavioral strategies focus on using verbal de-escalation, such as described by Richmond and colleagues,[17] to help the patient to calm and self-regulate his or her emotional state, and then allow the patient to begin to engage in his or her own treatment plan. The general approach consists of first helping the patient to feel safe by creating a nonthreatening environment, and speaking in calm, low tones. The interviewer attempting to engage with the patient should also be aware of the need for additional back up staff, should safety become a concern.[2,17] Working from an established rapport, the interviewer should then begin the discussion as to how to proceed with treatment. The interview should be concise, clear, and to the point. The interviewer should listen carefully to the patient and attempt to reach an understanding if possible. When discussing next treatments, it is helpful to lay out the range of options available and, if possible, allow the patient to choose. For instance, the interviewer may discuss that she would like to give the patient a medication to help him keep calm. The interviewer may then offer options, that is, would the patient rather try a pill or an injection. When the plan has been decided on, the provider should then review with the patient to gauge his or her understanding and engagement as an active participant in their own care.[17]

Suicidal Ideation

The first aspect of management of a patient with suicidal ideation is to find a safe place as the treatment location.[1] The decision of where to treat a suicidal patient depends on several factors. The range of settings includes a continuum of involuntary inpatient hospitalization to partial hospital and intensive outpatient programs to occasional ambulatory visits. Factors affecting this decision include (1) clinician's estimate of current suicide risk and potential for danger to others; (2) medical and psychiatric comorbidities; (3) strength and availability of psychosocial support network; and (4) ability to provide adequate self-care, give reliable feedback to the clinician, and cooperate with treatment.[4] A common tool used when the decision is made to treat in the outpatient setting is the no-harm contract. This contract should not be used as a substitute for careful clinical evaluation and should not be used with patients who are agitated, psychotic, impulsive, or under the influence of drugs or alcohol.[4] Once a treatment location is decided on, the patient and belongings should be searched for concealed weapons. In addition to weapons, the patient should be relieved of items with which they can cause self-harm. With active suicidal or homicidal ideation, 1:1 observation is useful and is commonly used.[1]

In the setting of depression, interpersonal psychotherapy and cognitive behavior therapy is appropriate. Additionally, cognitive behavioral therapy can decrease hopelessness and suicide attempts among patients in the outpatient setting. For patients with borderline personality disorder and suicidal ideation, psychodynamic therapy and dialectical behavior therapy may be useful.[4] Electroconvulsive therapy has proved useful in patients with suicidal ideation regardless of psychiatric diagnosis. It can even be used safely in pregnant women. Electroconvulsive therapy, however, is not enough for long-term maintenance. Thus electroconvulsive therapy should be done in combination with pharmacologic strategies. Finally, other strategies, such as rapid intervention, follow-up outreach, problem-solving therapy, brief psychological treatment, or group therapies, are thought to be useful despite limited evidence of efficacy.[4]

PHARMACOLOGIC STRATEGIES
Acute Psychosis, Mania, and Agitation or Homicidal Ideation

Should medications become necessary in the management of an acutely psychotic or agitated patient, there are numerous approaches, both general and specific. First-line approach for an agitated, but cooperative patient should consist of oral medications when possible. If rapid intervention or sedation is required, parenteral medications should be used.[15,16] A general approach to medications by suspected diagnosis, as proposed by consensus guidelines, is outlined in **Table 2** and **Box 6**.

In some cases when the agitated patient suffers from underlying medical comorbidities, it is important to adjust medications used and avoid others to prevent further complications. Benzodiazepines should be avoided in patients with chronic obstructive pulmonary disease, the elderly, and patients with known drug-seeking behavior or history of dependence and/or abuse. For patients with history of neurologic side effects, including akathisia, tardive dyskinesia, neuroleptic malignant syndrome, dystonia, or parkinsonian symptoms, typical antipsychotic medications should not be used (**Table 3**).[10]

Suicidal Ideation

The pharmacologic treatment of the patient with suicidal ideation depends on the psychiatric diagnosis. In general, evidence for the use of antidepressants is inconclusive for patients with suicidal ideation. Their proven benefits among patients with depressive episodes and anxiety are, however, in support of their use with suicidal patients. When using an antidepressant, it is preferable to use one with little risk of

Table 2
Pharmacologic treatments in psychiatric emergency

	Oral Medications		Parenteral Medications	
Suspected cause	First line	Second line	First line	Second line
Medical	None	TA BNZ	—	TA BNZ BNZ + AA
Substance				
Stimulant	BNZ	BNZ + TA TA	BNZ	BNZ + TA TA
Alcohol	—	BNZ	—	BNZ
Hallucinogen	—	BNZ BNZ + TA	BNZ	BNZ + TA
Opioids	None recommended		None recommended	
Primary psychiatric				
Unknown, no data	BNZ	BNZ + TA BNZ + AA	—	BNZ BNZ + TA
Schizophrenia	BNZ + TA BNZ + AA	Risperidone TA Olanzapine	BNZ + TA	TA
Mania	BNZ + TA BNZ + AA	BNZ TA Risperidone Olanzapine	BNZ + TA BNZ	TA
Depression with psychosis	—	BNZ + AA BNZ + TA BNZ Risperidone	BNZ + TA	BNZ
Personality disorder	—	BNZ	—	BNZ BNZ + TA
Posttraumatic stress disorder	BNZ	—	BNZ	BNZ + TA

Abbreviations: AA, atypical antipsychotic; BNZ, benzodiazepine; TA, typical antipsychotic.
Adapted from Allen MH, Currier GW, Hughes DH, et al. The expert consensus guideline series. Treatment of behavioral emergencies. Postgrad Med 2001;(Spec No):1–88; [quiz 89–90]; with permission.

lethality by means of an acute overdose. For this reason selective serotonin reuptake inhibitors or newer agents are preferable. For patients with insomnia, agitation, panic attacks, or psychic anxiety, benzodiazepines can be used on a short-term basis; however, when used, long-acting benzodiazepines are preferable and should be tapered. If benzodiazepines are not desired, other calming medications, such as trazadone, low doses of second-generation antipsychotics, and anticonvulsants can be used. There is evidence suggesting a benefit to the use of longer-term maintenance with lithium salts in reducing suicide and suicide attempts among patients with bipolar disorder and some evidence for use in major depressive disorder. Among patients with schizoaffective disorder, clozapine has demonstrated decreased suicide risk. However, with the risk of agranulocytosis and myocarditis, this medication should be reserved for those with frequent suicidal ideation or suicide attempts. Second-generation antipsychotics, such as risperidone, olanzapine, and quetiapine, are preferable to the first-generation antipsychotics.

> **Box 6**
> **Medications for agitation and psychosis**
>
> *Benzodiazepines*
> - Diazepam, 5–10 mg po q 30–60 minutes (average dose, 20–60 mg)
> - Lorazepam, 1–3 mg po or IM q 30–60 minutes
>
> *Typical Antipsychotics*
> - Haloperidol, 5–10 mg po or 5 mg IM every 30–60 minutes (average dose, 10–20 mg)
>
> *Atypical Antipsychotics*
> - Olanzapine, 5–10 mg po or 10 mg IM
> - Ziprasidone, 20–40 mg po bid or 10 mg IM q 2 hours or 20 mg IM q 4 hours
> - Risperidone, 2 mg po daily, increase by 1–2 mg q 24 hours until goal 4–8 mg; 25 mg IM q 2 weeks, start with po and continue oral for 3 weeks
> - Quetiapine, 25–50 mg po bid, increase by 25–50 mg bid until goal of 300–400 mg daily
>
> *Adapted from* Allen MH, Currier GW, Hughes DH, et al. The expert consensus guideline series. Treatment of behavioral emergencies. Postgrad Med 2001;(Spec No):1–88; [quiz 89–90]; with permission.

SELF-REGULATION STRATEGIES FOR PATIENTS

After any involuntary intervention with an agitated patient, it is the responsibility of the clinician who ordered such interventions to try to restore the therapeutic relationship and lessen the impact of any trauma from restraining interventions and prevent the risk

Table 3
Preferred medications for comorbid medical conditions

Medical Condition	Preferred Medication	Alternate Medication	Avoid
Chronic obstructive pulmonary disease	TA	AA	BNZ
Cardiac (arrhythmia or abnormal conduction)	BNZ	TA AA	—
Delirium	TA	AA	—
Dementia	AA TA	—	—
Elderly	AA	TA	BNZ
History of akathisia	BNZ AA	—	TA
History of tardive dyskinesia, neuroleptic malignant syndrome, dystonia, parkinsonian symptoms	BNZ	AA	TA
Mental retardation/developmental delay	AA	—	—
History for drug seeking, abuse, or dependence	—	AA TA	BNZ
History of seizures	BNZ	AA	—
Elevated blood alcohol and symptoms of withdraw	BNZ	—	—

Abbreviations: AA, atypical antipsychotic; BNZ, benzodiazepine; TA, typical antipsychotic.
  Adapted from Allen MH, Currier GW, Hughes DH, et al. The expert consensus guideline series. Treatment of behavioral emergencies. Postgrad Med 2001;(Spec No):1–88; [quiz 89–90]; with permission.

of additional violence. Clinicians should start by explaining why a restrictive intervention was necessary to the patient and the team. The team should explore alternatives for managing aggression if the patient were to get agitated again. If possible, the patient should be coached on how to request a time out and how to appropriately express his or her anger—using words, not physical force. Providers should explain how medications might help the patient feel calmer and prevent them from acting violently. Also, clinicians should continue to get the patient's feedback on whether his or her concerns have been addressed and then explain the plan, limitations, and expectations.

After the patient is calm, the clinician can acknowledge and work with the patient to help put the patient's concerns into perspective, and assist him or her in problem solving the initial precipitating situation. Because prevention of agitation is the best way to treat it, planning with the patient is best: "What works when you are very upset as you were today? What can we/you do in the future to help you stay in control?"[17]

DEBRIEFING AND TEAM-MANAGEMENT STRATEGIES

Managing a psychiatric emergency is emotionally and mentally taxing for patients, family and friends, and the health care team. It is therefore important to debrief with all, including the patient's family, who witnessed the incident. The debriefing should include the following themes:

- Common reactions
  - Fear of one's own emotional reaction
  - Fear of patient's emotional reaction
  - Fear of being blamed for bad news
  - Fear of not knowing all the answers
  - Fear of the patient's suffering/death
  - Fear of one's own mortality or that of a loved one
  - Feeling of having failed or being powerless
- Identify your feelings
- Share your reactions with a trusted colleague or mentor
- Consider writing about your reactions
- Participate in restoring rituals or strategies

If restraint or force needs to be used, it is important that the health care team be debriefed on the actions after the event. Staff should feel free to suggest what went well during the episode, and what did not, and recommend improvements for the next episode.[20,21]

LEGAL CONSIDERATIONS

There are special legal considerations concerning patients with psychiatric emergencies. The 1975 US Supreme Court ruling in the case of *O'Conner v Donaldson* gave persons with mental illness rights when it came to involuntary admission. This ruling indicated that mental illness alone was not sufficient for an involuntary admission.[1,11] Following this ruling, states also restricted the involuntary admission to a predetermined time period of days to weeks after which time the patient was entitled to a court hearing to determine if the involuntary admission should continue. This time is commonly 72 hours and often known as the 72-hour hold (**Box 7**).[1,11]

In response to these criteria, the American Psychiatric Association developed a model in which a patient must meet all six criteria to be eligible for involuntary admission: (1) mental illness, (2) danger to self or others, (3) refusal to consent,

---

Box 7
Criteria for involuntary admissions

1. Mental illness
2. Danger to self or others
3. Refusal to consent
4. Treatability
5. Lack capacity to make treatment decisions
6. Hospitalization is least restrictive treatment

From Sood TR, McStay CM. Evaluation of the psychiatric patient. Emerg Med Clin North Am 2009;27(4):669–83, ix; with permission.

---

(4) treatability, (5) lack the capacity to make treatment decisions, and (6) hospitalization as the least restrictive treatment.[1] To commit a patient, the physician has to complete an initial certificate and hold the patient in a psychiatric facility until further legal proceedings. When completing a petition for involuntary admission, the clinician should make three copies for (1) medical record, (2) ambulance/police, and (3) hospital records. Then the physician has 72 hours to hold a hearing for involuntary hospitalization or the patient is allowed to leave. Involuntary commitment statutes vary from state to state, thus it is important for clinicians to be aware of the statutes and processes in their jurisdiction.[1]

For patients with homicidal ideation, clinicians should be aware of civil commitment laws in their jurisdiction. In some jurisdictions, physicians are legally responsible for informing the potential victim and/or the police.[1]

SUMMARY/DISCUSSION

The American Psychiatric Association defines a psychiatric emergency as "an acute disturbance in thought, behavior, mood, or social relationship, which requires immediate intervention as defined by the patient, family, or social unit." These diagnoses, which require immediate intervention to save the patient and/or others from imminent danger, include mania, acute psychosis, suicidal ideation, and homicidal ideation. The evaluation of patients exhibiting psychiatric emergencies starts by ensuring safety for all, then proceeding with evaluation. It is also important to determine if there is a comorbid medical diagnosis or a medical diagnosis causing the symptoms. The management of psychiatric emergencies is first dependent on whether the patient is a potential harm to themselves or others. This and other factors affecting urgency determine the treatment location. Specific management of the patient then ultimately depends on the cause of the psychiatric symptoms. Medications used focus first on calming the patient and then treating the disease. The range of therapy modalities also depend on cause. After dealing with psychiatric emergencies, it is important to debrief with the patient and family to help ensure a continued effective therapeutic relationship. Additionally, it is important to debrief with the health care team about how the situation was handled. It is also important to debrief with providers and staff to help restore mental health because psychiatric emergencies are emotionally taxing for all involved. Finally, there are important legal considerations that a clinician must be aware of, particularly in the setting of involuntary admission. Providers should be aware of their local jurisdiction's individual requirements. Psychiatric emergencies in medical settings are frequent in hospital and outpatient settings. Therefore, primary care medical providers, including nursing and support staff, need to be trained in the assessment, treatment, and management of these patients.

REFERENCES

1. Sood TR, McStay CM. Evaluation of the psychiatric patient. Emerg Med Clin North Am 2009;27(4):669–83, ix.
2. Mavrogiorgou P, Brune M, Juckel G. The management of psychiatric emergencies. Dtsch Arztebl Int 2011;108(13):222–30.
3. Feldman MD, Franks P, Duberstein PR, et al. Let's not talk about it: suicide inquiry in primary care. Ann Fam Med 2007;5(5):412–8.
4. Practice guideline for the assessment and treatment of patients with suicidal behaviors. Am J Psychiatry 2003;160(11 Suppl):1–60.
5. Pilowsky DJ, Olfson M, Gameroff MJ, et al. Panic disorder and suicidal ideation in primary care. Depress Anxiety 2006;23(1):11–6.
6. Schulberg HC, Bruce ML, Lee PW, et al. Preventing suicide in primary care patients: the primary care physician's role. Gen Hosp Psychiatry 2004;26(5):337–45.
7. Bartels SJ, Coakley E, Oxman TE, et al. Suicidal and death ideation in older primary care patients with depression, anxiety, and at-risk alcohol use. Am J Geriatr Psychiatry 2002;10(4):417–27.
8. Williams AJ. Fatal self-harm in the elderly. Med Sci Law 2002;42(1):87 [author reply: 87–8].
9. Pirkis JE, Burgess PM, Johnston AK, et al. Use of selective serotonin reuptake inhibitors and suicidal ideation: findings from the 2007 National Survey of Mental Health and Wellbeing. Med J Aust 2010;192(1):53.
10. Allen MH, Currier GW, Hughes DH, et al. The Expert Consensus Guideline Series. Treatment of behavioral emergencies. Postgrad Med 2001;(Spec No): 1–88 [quiz: 89–90].
11. Testa M, West SG. Civil commitment in the United States. Psychiatry (Edgmont) 2010;7(10):30–40.
12. Huff JS, Farace E, Brady WJ, et al. The quick confusion scale in the ED: comparison with the mini-mental state examination. Am J Emerg Med 2001;19(6):461–4.
13. Corrigan JD. Development of a scale for assessment of agitation following traumatic brain injury. J Clin Exp Neuropsychol 1989;11(2):261–77.
14. Zun LS. Pitfalls in the care of the psychiatric patient in the emergency department. J Emerg Med 2012;43(5):829–35.
15. Slade M, Taber D, Clarke MM, et al. Best practices for the treatment of patients with mental and substance use illnesses in the emergency department. Dis Mon 2007;53(11–12):536–80.
16. Lukens TW, Wolf SJ, Edlow JA, et al. Clinical policy: critical issues in the diagnosis and management of the adult psychiatric patient in the emergency department. Ann Emerg Med 2006;47(1):79–99.
17. Richmond JS, Berlin JS, Fishkind AB, et al. Verbal de-escalation of the agitated patient: consensus statement of the American Association for Emergency Psychiatry Project BETA De-escalation Workgroup. West J Emerg Med 2012;13(1): 17–25.
18. Kennedy GJ, Onuogu E, Lowinger R. Psychiatric emergencies: rapid response and life-saving therapies. Geriatrics 1999;54(9):38–42, 45–6.
19. Bernert RA, Hom MA, Roberts LW. A review of multidisciplinary clinical practice guidelines in suicide prevention: toward an emerging standard in suicide risk

assessment and management, training and practice. Acad Psychiatry 2014; 38(5):585–92.

20. Dyregrov A. The process in psychological debriefings. J Trauma Stress 1997; 10(4):589–605.

21. Flannery RB Jr. The Assaulted Staff Action Program (ASAP): common issues in fielding a team. Psychiatr Q 1998;69(2):135–42.

Physician Wellness Across the Professional Spectrum

Russell Blackwelder, MD, MDiv*, Kristen Hood Watson, MD, John R. Freedy, MD, PhD

KEYWORDS

- Wellness • Burnout • Physician well-being • Career stage and health

KEY POINTS

- Physician wellness continues to be an area of growing concern for health systems, particularly as it relates to primary care physicians.
- Wellness and burnout continue to have major impacts on individual physicians and their families, and on the health system as a whole.
- Strategies exist to help physicians to cope with career stresses as studies continue to accumulate pertaining to awareness regarding physician wellness and burnout.

INTRODUCTION

Physician wellness has emerged as a key concern. Debates, followed by changes to medical and resident education, have taken place in recent years, not the least of which has been restriction of duty hours. When new physicians stand and recite the Hippocratic Oath today, with many schools using the modern oath, these doctors pledge "an awareness of my own frailty."[1]

However, this pledge has proven easier said than upheld. The culture of medicine and the journey through training frequently put the health and well-being of the physician last, with competencies in training for residents that require demonstration of "responsiveness to patient needs that supersedes self-interest."[2] Frequently, the care of self falls to the bottom of the list in the midst of the day's demands, particularly for primary care physicians as they balance the workload of patients and their families, paperwork, referrals, and administrative upkeep. The impact of diminished wellness among physicians has been associated with everything from patients' health and safety, to successful health care reform.[3]

Wallace and colleagues[4] have argued that physician wellness has risen to a level of importance for societal systems and the population, and that it should now also be

Disclosure Statement: The authors have nothing to disclose.
Department of Family Medicine, Medical University of South Carolina, 9228 Medical Plaza Drive, Charleston, SC 29406, USA
* Corresponding author.
E-mail address: blackwr@musc.edu

among the many quality indicators that are present in medicine. The Accreditation Council of Graduate Medical Education (ACGME) has also placed heightened interest in recent years on the topic of wellness among physicians.[5] This increased attention is most notable in the ACGME's Clinical Learning Environment Review, which has set forth guidelines for programs to educate trainees regarding burnout and also to assess its impact among residents.[6] Some medical schools even prepare classes to address such topics as "How to avoid suicide."[7] This article provides an overview of wellness and burnout among physicians across the spectrum of professional life — medical student, postgraduate trainee, and various stages of the doctor's career — and highlight strategies shown to strengthen the physician's very real frailty.

> Burnout can be defined as "a maladaptive syndrome that results from chronic work stress...and characterized by feeling emotionally depleted (emotional exhaustion) and/or having a distant or uncaring attitude toward patients and work (depersonalization or cynicism)."

WELLNESS AND BURNOUT

Burnout has been described as the antithesis of wellness, as argued by McClafferty and Brown.[8] Burnout is measured most often with the Maslach Burnout Inventory, which specifically addresses 3 components: emotional exhaustion, depersonalization, and low sense of personal accomplishment (**Box 1**). The first 2 components of this scale are most frequently areas of poor scoring among physicians.[9] Burnout is further defined as "a maladaptive syndrome that results from chronic work stress...and characterized by feeling emotionally depleted (emotional exhaustion) and/or having a distant or uncaring attitude toward patients and work (depersonalization or cynicism)," according to Jennings and Slavin.[6] Overall, the literature suggests that burnout effects anywhere from 30% to 40% of physicians,[10] and even up to 75%. Compared with the general population, physicians are more likely to commit suicide, and burnout contributes to the 8% to 12% rate of substance abuse among physicians.[11] With health care reform increasing the numbers of patients with access to care, the increasing rate of administrative oversight, and loss of autonomy for many physicians, the future remains unclear as to how these numbers might be affected.

In contrast, wellness has been defined as "the complex and multifaceted nature of physicians' physical, mental and emotional health and well-being."[10] Many aspects are in the purview of wellness, but frequently noted is the idea of resiliency, which includes self-awareness, self-care, and maintenance of values. Brennan and McGrady[2] argue that, despite this quality being traditionally thought of as an immutable one, resiliency can actually be taught and enhanced. According to the authors, the domains of resiliency include insight, self-care, and values. Areas that have been shown to improve physician wellness are work–life balance, social support, adequate rest, and regular physical activity.[8] Presently, the bulk of research and data that have

---

Box 1
Components of the Maslach burnout inventory

Emotional exhaustion

Depersonalization

Low sense of personal accomplishment

accumulated in the field has focused on the area of burnout, and fewer studies have sought to expand on the topic of preventive strategies and ways to improve well-being.[6]

Wellness has been defined as "the complex and multifaceted nature of physicians' physical, mental and emotional health and well-being."

CAREER STAGE AND WELLNESS
Medical School

As learners are beginning to accumulate medical knowledge and the ability to manage patients, they are also beginning to accumulate higher rates of burnout than the general population when matched for age. The prevalence of depression and anxiety are anywhere from 25% to greater than 50%.[12] Specifically, burnout affects up to 50% of United States medical students. Reports indicate that anywhere from 3% to 15% of medical students have suicidal ideation during their time in medical school.[13] Dyrbye and colleagues[14] were able to show the professional effects of such burnout in a study published in 2010. In that study, students from 7 medical schools who were experiencing symptoms of burnout were more likely to engage in self-reported unprofessional behavior and were also less likely to experience thoughts of altruism. Additionally, levels of burnout seem to correlate with thoughts of dropping out of medical school, which may lead to great debt, loss of time investment, and alteration of career plans, if carried out.[15]

Residency

Residency is a time of intense training and work demands, as young physicians bear increasing responsibility. Studies of postgraduate trainees from all specialties reveal that more than one-half have experienced depressive symptoms and more than 8% have had suicidal thoughts over the preceding 12 months.[6] Studies of residents place the rates of burnout between 27% and 75%. Even after duty-hour restrictions were put in place, family medicine residents had scores consistent with burnout in the range of 14% to 24%. At the same time, behaviors known to be protective of burnout such as exercise, adequate sleep, and healthy diets were only present in 20% to 25% of family medicine residents.[2] As medical school debt continues to increase, today's residents face the additional financial stress that the system of medical education is largely unfamiliar with. In the past 20 years, medical school debt has tripled, with 2012 graduates entering residency with a median medical school debt of $170,000 (**Box 2**).[6] This burden certainly continues into early professional life after graduate medical education training is complete.

Box 2
Medical school debt in 2012

- 52% of male residents and 43% female residents feel unfairly compensated.

- 86% graduate with medical school debt.

- Median medical school debt = $170,000

Data from Jennings ML, Slavin SJ. Resident wellness matters: optimizing resident education and wellness through the learning environment. Acad Med 2015;90(9):1–5.

Practicing Physicians

In a study by Dyrbye and colleagues,[9] 7288 physicians were surveyed and classified as early career (≤10 years of practice), midcareer (11–20 years of practice), and late career (≥21 years of practice). Their findings revealed that midcareer physicians had higher rates of emotional exhaustion and overall burnout, whereas depersonalization was highest among early career doctors but decreased as careers advanced (**Table 1**). The higher levels of burnout among those in midcareer persisted even when adjusted for practice type, sex, and specialty. Satisfaction with practicing medicine as a career was lowest for early career doctors and increased throughout the stages of a career. Specifically, career satisfaction was lowest for primary care specialties and in surgeons in the first 10 years of their career. Of note, middle career physicians were more likely to consider changing their practice venue or leaving medicine altogether out of frustration.

RECOGNITION

The first step in regaining physician wellness is to recognize that there is a problem. This can be achieved through several methods: self-identification, colleague identification, or through hospital or other governing bodies. Unfortunately, the idea that physicians should "tough it out"[16] with regard to stress and depression seems to be cultivated as early as during medical school training. Therefore, an important initial step is to educate physicians, and those who are in the position of monitoring physician well-being, on what constitutes signs of burnout, depression, or other types of impairment. Understanding what is considered to be an abnormal amount of stress and that, in fact, there is such a thing as too much stress, may help physicians to recognize their own signs of burnout. Additionally, it may help physicians to identify their colleagues who need assistance.

Traditionally, the notion of "The Triple Aim" has been used as a guide for health care organizations to be highly functional and successful. Bodenheimer and Sinksy have suggested that it is time to move from the triple aim theory to a "quadruple aim," inclusive of concern for the work life of health care providers.[17] In short, they argue that although the focus continues to include enhancing patient experience, improving population health, and reducing costs (the triple aims), it is also time for health care systems to include the goal of enhancing the well-being of its providers.[17]

DESTIGMATIZE

If physicians are worried about their professional livelihood, in addition to their already present stressors, they may be less likely to seek help. Also, physician coworkers may

Table 1
Burnout at various stages

Career Stage	Definition	Finding
Early career	First 10 y of practice	1. Most likely dissatisfied with medicine as career choice. 2. Most likely to experience depersonalization.
Midcareer	11–20 y of practice	1. Most likely to experience burnout and emotional exhaustion. 2. Most likely to consider job change, including leaving patient care.
Late career	≥21 y of practice	—

Adapted from Dyrbye LN, Varkey P, Boone SL, et al. Physician satisfaction and burnout at different career stages. Mayo Clin Proc 2013;88(12):1358–67.

not want to harm their friends by reporting them. Although substance abuse among physicians is discussed more commonly and seems to have a clearer strategy for treatment, other areas of impairment are less well-defined. The prevailing notion that physicians cannot admit flaws and therefore must suffer in silence remains. The American Medical Association reports that all physicians should have their own personal physician and that, unless there is a concern that a practicing doctor is too impaired to see patients, the Health Insurance Portability and Accountability Act applies and privacy should be maintained.[18] A study from San Diego School of Medicine helped to destigmatize burnout by providing educational lectures. At that institution, 83% of departments participated in the lectures and several requested further education on the topic of physician burnout and suicide.[16]

SCREENING

If there are no clear signs of impairment that may be picked up by a colleague or supervisor, what else can be done? One study at the University of California San Diego (UCSD), completed by Moutier and colleagues,[16] found that screening may be effective for identifying medical professionals at risk of suicide. The study looked at anonymous screening of medical and pharmacy students, residents, and faculty. Based on the screening results, the participants were provided with interpretation from a counselor and then offered a referral as indicated.

Screening large numbers of participants would be difficult unless made mandatory. The Moutier study, for example, had a 13% response rate. Also, if there is an associated stigma, the questions may not be answered honestly. This study helped to mitigate that issue by keeping the survey anonymous even if suicidality was present.

In the UCSD study, 94% surveyed were considered to be at moderate to high risk of suicide with 27% in the high-risk category. Despite respondents having access to the counselor, whether online, by phone, or in person, and being offered referral for further evaluation, the follow-up was limited. In the most concerning group, only 17% accepted the referral for additional evaluation.[16]

METHODS FOR IMPROVEMENT

In a 2015 survey by Cejka Search,[19] 65% of physician respondents reported concerns about work–life balance. Possible solutions offered included flexible full-time work schedules, shared positions, and part-time positions. Physician Wellness Services and Cejka Search published results from their 2011 survey that allowed physicians to comment on ways to decrease stress and burnout. As mentioned with the 2015 survey, better work hours were the most commonly cited method (32.5%). Work–life balance was number two. Other methods of improving physician wellness included improving finances, making time for self-care, and increasing support with administrative tasks at work.[20]

Previous articles noted that an increase in physician happiness was correlated with having a positive attitude and/or religious belief system, being in a relationship or having strong social support, and receiving positive feedback. One qualitative analysis investigated how physicians can improve their own well-being. The physicians were surveyed to find out the practices they use to promote self-wellness. The primary methods of wellness promotion included having a generally positive approach to life, maintaining relationships, pursuing spiritual/religious involvement, participating in self-care activities (ie, healthy diet, exercise, counseling), and finding fulfillment in work life (**Box 3**). There was a trend among all toward increased physician well-being, but the only statistically significant method ($P<.01$) was the general approach to life.[21]

Box 3
Methods of wellness promotion

Generally positive approach to life[a]

Maintaining relationships

Spiritual/religious involvement

Participating in self-care activities (healthy diet, exercise, counseling)

Fulfilling work life

[a] Statistically significant.
Adapted from Weiner EL. A qualitative study of physician's own wellness-promotion practices. West J Med 2001;174:19–23.

FUTURE GOALS

To improve the focus on physician wellness, buy in from the health care organization or leadership may be the most advantageous place to start. Although physicians can, of course, work on decreasing stress levels, many may be caught up in their current circumstances and be unable to see the alternatives. If a workplace offered education and possibly screening regarding wellness, as mentioned, recognition of issues and targeting of resources for improvement could be linked.

One benefit to organizations would include less turnover, which means less money spent on recruiting. Fewer vacant positions would likely lead to less work pressure on the remaining physicians. In addition, happier physicians would likely create a better overall work environment, which would be beneficial to the whole office. Of note, prior articles on physician wellness indicate that providers with a compromised state of wellness may provide a lower quality of care.[18] This could also be associated with decreased patient satisfaction. Concerns about patient care should be reason enough for an institution to want to improve physician well-being. Ideally, there is also value placed on the happiness and success of the employees.

SUMMARY

Physician wellness is an area of growing interest as more attention is placed on rigorous demands of training and practice throughout a physician's career. With rates of burnout, depression, suicide, and substance abuse at high levels among doctors, the focus will remain increased as solutions are sought to improve the well-being of those called to this form of service in society. Particularly for primary care physicians who maintain such close relationships with patients and engage in such a wide variety of activities, the importance of not only maintaining, but also enhancing, wellness will remain an issue of utmost importance.

REFERENCES

1. More about the modern Hippocratic oath. John Hopkins University Library. Available at: http://guides.library.jhu.edu/c.php?g=202502&p=1335759. Accessed August 27, 2015.
2. Brennan J, McGrady A. Designing and implementing a resiliency program for family medicine residents. Int J Psychiatry Med 2015;50(1):104–14.
3. Dyrbye LN, Shanafelt TD. Physician burnout: a potential threat to successful health care reform. JAMA 2011;305(19):2009–10.

4. Wallace JE, Lemaire JB, Ghali WA. Physician wellness: a missing quality indicator. Lancet 2009;374:1714–21.
5. Vassar L. ACGME seeks to transform residency to foster wellness. 2015. Available at: http://www.ama-assn.org/ama/ama-wire/post/acgme-seeks-transform-residency-foster-wellness. Accessed July 28, 2015.
6. Jennings ML, Slavin SJ. Resident wellness matters: optimizing resident education and wellness through the learning environment. Acad Med 2015;90(9):1–5.
7. Devi S. Doctors in distress. Lancet 2011;377:454–5.
8. McClafferty H, Brown OW. Physician health and wellness. Pediatrics 2014;134(4):830–5.
9. Dyrbye LN, Varkey P, Boone SL, et al. Physician satisfaction and burnout at different career stages. Mayo Clin Proc 2013;88(12):1358–67.
10. Siedsma M, Emle L. Physician burnout: can we make a difference together? Crit Care 2015;19(1):273.
11. Doctors get ill too. Lancet 2009;374:1653.
12. Dunn LB, Iglewicz A, Moutier C. A conceptual model of medical student well-being: promoting resilience and preventing burnout. Acad Psychiatry 2008;32(1):44–53.
13. Dyrbye LN, Thomas MR, Massie FS, et al. Burnout and suicidal ideation among U.S. medical students. Ann Intern Med 2008;149:334–41.
14. Dyrbye LN, Massie FS, Eacker A, et al. Relationship between burnout and professional conduct and attitudes among US medical students. JAMA 2010;301(11):1173–80.
15. Dyrbye LN, Thomas MR, Power DV, et al. Burnout and serious thoughts of dropping out of medical school: a multi-institutional study. Acad Med 2010;85(1):94–102.
16. Moutier C, Norcross W, Jong P, et al. The suicide prevention and depression awareness program at the University of California, San Diego School of Medicine. Acad Med 2012;87:320–6.
17. Bodenheimer T, Sinsky C. From the triple to quadruple aim: care of the patient requires care of the provider. Ann Fam Med 2014;12(6):573–6.
18. Taub S, Morin K, Goldrich MS, et al, Council on Ethical and Judicial Affairs of the American Medical Association. Physician health and wellness. Occup Med 2006;56(2):77–82.
19. Physician stress and burnout at all-time high! How to stop the bleeding & create an environment for improved physician engagement. Cejka Search; 2015.
20. Physician stress and burnout survey: executive summary. 2011.
21. Weiner EL. A qualitative study of physician's own wellness-promotion practices. West J Med 2001;174:19–23.

Moving?

Make sure your subscription moves with you!

To notify us of your new address, find your **Clinics Account Number** (located on your mailing label above your name), and contact customer service at:

Email: journalscustomerservice-usa@elsevier.com

800-654-2452 (subscribers in the U.S. & Canada)
314-447-8871 (subscribers outside of the U.S. & Canada)

Fax number: 314-447-8029

Elsevier Health Sciences Division
Subscription Customer Service
3251 Riverport Lane
Maryland Heights, MO 63043

*To ensure uninterrupted delivery of your subscription, please notify us at least 4 weeks in advance of move.

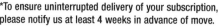